Raymond M. Costello, Ph. D.
Department of Psychiatry
University of Texas
OC Medical School at San Antonio
7703 Floyd Curl Drive
San Antonio, Texas 78229

Behavior Therapy in Clinical Psychiatry

Behavior Therapy in Clinical Psychiatry

V. Meyer and Edward S. Chesser

SCIENCE HOUSE, INC.
NEW YORK

Copyright © V. Meyer and Edward S. Chesser, 1970

Library of Congress Catalog Card Number: 71-159480
Standard Book Number: 87668-043-0

Manufactured in the United States of America

Contents

Editorial Foreword

Behaviour therapy is at once among the newest forms of treatment in psychiatry – and one of the oldest: sticks and carrots have always been used to modify human behaviour.

The fundamental assumption of behaviour therapy is that the patient, having previously been well and having now become ill, i.e. now manifesting disturbed behaviour, can be seen as having 'acquired' new patterns of behaviour. In a general sense we can see the change as like that which results from learning; and, in common speech, what can be learned can be unlearned. The assumption is supported by experimental evidence, for it has been proved that under given circumstances we can produce abnormalities of behaviour in animals analagous to those human disturbances which we call mental illness. The difference between behaviour therapy and traditional methods of reward and punishment lies in the former's detailed knowledge and understanding of the precise conditions under which behaviour can be modified.

Even if we believe that mental illness is based fundamentally on physiological and biochemical changes in the person, we cannot ignore the fact that such disease processes can manifest themselves only through the changing of acquired patterns of behaviour which are normal for that individual in his social circumstances. We can, therefore, apply the principles of learning to modify the patient's behaviour in such a way as to minimize the changes produced by the underlying hypothetical disturbances.

Put in this general way the principles of behaviour therapy seem little more than common sense; almost platitudinous and certainly innocuous. Why then should there be so much controversy about behaviour therapy, which has raised such an uproar that it has spread far beyond the worlds of psychiatry and psychology? (And I leave aside the fierce debates as to its moral justification.) The reason is because it cuts out all those theories about the dynamic unconscious, unconscious mechanisms, symbolism and psychosexual development which underlie much current thinking, ranging from psychoanalysis to existentialism, about mental illness. Behaviour therapy, therefore, challenges current ideas which have exerted immense influence, not only in psychiatry and psychology but in the arts and journalism as well. Behaviour therapy also differs from them, as the authors modestly point out, in that it makes no claim to account for the totality of the human psyche.

The authors describe the principles of conditioning and learning, and consider impartially the relation between current practice in behaviour therapy and those principles. Where there is no such relationship, they say so, openly. Behaviour therapy is very new and it is therefore not surprising that the exploration of new techniques should leave theory behind. This is a common experience in the early stages of the applied sciences: theory is inadequate but serves as a jumping-off point for the development of techniques and these, in turn, lead to the modification of theory.

The authors have written a cogent account of 'the state of the art'; their description of behaviour therapy is one of the most succinct in the literature, yet nothing has been sacrificed for the sake of brevity. Finally, the writing is so clear that even those who approach the subject for the first time will have no difficulty in understanding it. The authors confirm in this book their reputation for their contribution both to the theory and to the practice of behaviour therapy.

MAX HAMILTON

Chapter 1   Introduction

The causes of human behaviour have interested man from the dawn of civilization. The psychologist or psychiatrist has no monopoly in this subject, which falls within the experience of everyone. It is said that we are all psychologists in the sense of wishing to understand, predict and control the behaviour of ourselves and others. It seems to be inherent in human nature to want to understand all phenomena, and a wealth of explanatory systems, from magic to atomic radiation, bears witness to this need. To maintain a neutral attitude towards any theory until observable data have been adequately described requires much discipline, for 'we are born with expectations'. The more complex the subject matter, the greater the profusion of theories and hypotheses; compare the frugality of physics in its use of theories with the extravagance of the behavioural sciences. As phenomena become more accurately described and measured, the number and diversity of explanatory theories diminish.

In this book we present an account of the theoretical basis, methods, clinical application and efficacy of behaviour therapy in psychiatry, a therapy which claims derivation from modern learning theory. There is also a description of recent research findings of relevance to the validity of behaviour therapy theory and the identification of the effective processes of psychological treatment. In this chapter a brief outline is given of the subject matter of psychiatry, together with some of its commonly used concepts and treatment methods, to serve as a background for the discussion of behaviour therapy. Obviously, no attempt has been made to make this outline comprehensive in breadth or in depth, but it may be of some help to those unfamiliar with clinical psychiatry.

Most definitions of psychiatric disorder state that its chief manifestation is abnormal behaviour, a term which includes subjective experience. Normality is a concept used in two different senses, the statistical and the ideal. The statistical norm is the average or usual, whilst deviation from the mean is designated abnormal. There is no necessary value judgement attached to this concept of normality. The genius and the idiot are both abnormal by this criterion. The ideal norm refers to that which is most desirable. There can be considerable divergencies of opinion on what constitutes ideal normality, whereas statistical normality is a more objective criterion. However, there are certain difficulties involved in determining statistical normality, particularly in the constitution of the sample population. For example, in the assessment of patterns of behaviour, such factors as age, sex, intelligence, social and cultural background may need to be taken into consideration. Behaviour which is normal for a Samoan child would be found to be outside the range of normal behaviour for a London bank manager.

In clinical practice most psychiatrists employ the statistical concept of normality in their assessment of behaviour, and then attempt to ascertain whether any abnormal behaviour is causing suffering to the individual or others in his environment. Behaviour that is both abnormal and causes suffering is sufficient to indicate the presence of 'mental (psychiatric) disorder' in the opinion of some psychiatrists. Such a definition encompasses the persistently naughty child or the habitual criminal as well as the bizarre behaviour of a deluded patient. However, some psychiatrists take into consideration the supposed causes of the behaviour, as well as the behaviour itself, before diagnosing 'mental disorder'.

Disease is an abstract concept, and can therefore be fashioned according to one's choice. The most simple model of a disease is one in which a specific cause initiates a specific pattern of symptoms which follow a predictable course and which are associated with specific structural or functional changes in particular parts of the body (somatic pathology). In practice, few diseases can be defined in this way because there is rarely such perfect correlation between cause, symptoms, course and demonstrable pathology. The causes are often uncertain and there may be no demonstrable somatic pathology. Because of this some diseases are delineated on the basis of clinical symptomatology only, whereas others are classified on the basis of established or presumptive aetiology or pathology. One commonly canvassed view of disease is to restrict the term to conditions associated with demonstrable somatic pathology, at the same time accepting the possibility or probability that advances in technique will lead to the discovery of somatic changes in some of the disorders in which none have so far been detected.

The notion of 'mental illness' and its differentiation from disorders of behaviour and variations in personality remains a contentious subject (e.g. Jaspers, 1963; Lewis, 1953; Szasz, 1961). Despite lack of agreement on this topic, it is still possible and desirable to use a system of classification which is operationally defined (for recent reviews see Stengel, 1959; Zubin, 1967; General Register Office, 1968). Related to the problem of the delineation and classification of psychiatric disorders is the problem of deciding what constitutes a 'symptom'. This is of practical importance in the assessment of the effects of psychiatric treatment. In such an assessment the patient is likely to be concerned with both physical and psychological symptoms such as pain or anxiety and his level of social, sexual and occupational adjustment, whether or not psychiatrists regard them as symptoms, defence mechanisms, or determined by personality or social variables. A patient may be reassured to hear that his anxiety or depression or gambling is not due to any disease but he may still find it unwelcome and be pleased if it could be modified or eliminated. The many attempts to define 'mental health' and 'mental illness' bear witness to the difficulty of the task (Lewis, 1953). It is not possible to draw a distinction between disorders of behaviour and psychiatric disorder with any degree of confidence. Attempts are made on the basis of inferred psychological processes or descriptive criteria in terms of the persistence and inappropriateness of the behaviour and the suffering which accompanies it. Some writers consider that psychiatric symptoms can be acquired through ordinary learning processes (e.g. Wolpe, 1958) while others specifically exclude learned behaviour (Hebb, 1947).

Some types of abnormal behaviour are found to be associated with observable somatic disorder, structural, biochemical or electrical, in the brain or other parts of the body. It is usual to classify these under the heading of 'organic psychiatric (mental) disorders'. The causes of the pathological changes are as varied as those found in other bodily diseases and include, for example, injuries, infections and tumours. The actual psychological symptoms present in a particular patient depend more on the site, duration and severity of the cerebral damage than its cause. Even in these organic disorders, pre-existing personality traits, intelligence level and the social environment of the patient may have a significant influence on the symptomatology.

The cardinal symptoms of the organic disorders are clouding of consciousness, which may vary from slight drowsiness to deep coma, together with impairment of recent memory and disorientation in place and time. This behavioural disturbance is usually found in association with some somatic pathology, although it is difficult to predict accurately the severity and type of symptoms from a knowledge of the structural damage alone. Nonetheless, it would be reasonable to consider the somatic disturbance as one cause of the abnormal behaviour. For example, the drowsiness and forgetfulness of a patient with an extensive brain tumour may be said to be caused by the brain tumour. The organic psychiatric disorders therefore exemplify a group of conditions which are pathological disease entities with abnormal behaviour as one manifestation. In a limited sense at least, one cause of the abnormal behaviour is known.

Psychiatric disorders are more often found to be unassociated with detectable somatic disorder and causation is uncertain. They are therefore referred to, provisionally at least, as 'functional psychiatric disorders'. The commonly used classification of these conditions is a descriptive one according to symptomatology and course. They can be subdivided into two large categories, psychotic and neurotic. The distinction is not clear-cut, but is based on the severity of the disorder, the degree of social disability it causes and the degree of insight present. The psychotic disorders correspond to the lay concept of insanity and may include such manifestations as delusions, hallucinations and an inability to distinguish between fantasy and reality.

Two main forms of functional psychosis are recognized, manic-depressive, in which the main symptom is a disorder of mood such as persistent elation or depression, and schizophrenia, in which there is disorganization of the individual's personality with disturbances of feeling and thinking. The other large subgroup of functional disorders, the non-psychotic, include the neuroses and the personality disorders. In this group there is considerable controversy over classification and aetiology. The neuroses are usually classified according to the main symptoms – anxiety, phobic, depressive, obsessive-compulsive or hysterical reactions, but mixed forms are common. Personality disorder is a descriptive term applied to those people who have recurrent life-long difficulties, either in the form of subjective symptoms such as anxiety or depression, or in their ability to make satisfactory interpersonal relationships in family and social life or work. This latter group includes the solitary, the paranoid and the immature personalities as well as the antisocial psychopath. People who have personality disorders may, in addition, develop an acute neurotic reaction or a psychosis more frequently than those with normal personalities.

Theories of psychiatric disorders

The classification above is a descriptive one based on symptoms and course. Inevitably, in our present state of knowledge, theories of aetiology of the 'functional disorders' reflect our uncertainty. It is a truism to state that the causes of abnormal behaviour are multiple and will include both hereditary and environmental factors. Hereditary factors have been demonstrated most clearly in some of the less common organic disorders (some types of mental deficiency and dementia). There is reasonably good evidence of a genetic influence in the psychoses, and some evidence in the neuroses and personality disorders. What is actually inherited is not clear, but both physical characteristics such as body build and the psychological structure of personality appear to be under genetic influence and tend to correlate with each other. It used to be thought that a general predisposition to mental illness or moral weakness, which was labelled 'degeneracy', was inherited. Modern genetic views favour the theory of a more specific inheritance of particular psychiatric diseases. A comparatively recent finding has been the association of certain chromosomal abnormalities with low intelligence and personality disorder. The physiological and psychological mechanisms which bring this about are unknown.

Introduction

The environmental factors which may help to fashion the behaviour of the individual and any 'disease' he may suffer will, in theory, include his whole life experience from conception onwards. Physical, psychological and social influences combine to furnish a unique environment for each individual. For this reason Adolf Meyer saw psychiatric disorder as a unique reaction of an individual to his environment. The shortest diagnostic label would be the patient's name.

Theorists have ranged widely in their search for the environmental causes of mental disorder. When psychiatry emerged from its Dark Age, in which mental disorder was attributed to divine or demoniacal possession or wickedness and fell within the province of the theologian or philosopher rather than the physician, there was a return to the Hippocratic teaching that the brain was the seat of the mind, and madness was due to disorder of the brain brought about by natural causes. 'Mental diseases are brain diseases' became the fashionable slogan and the discovery of their somatic pathology was confidently expected. For the majority of mental disorders this demonstration is still awaited, with varying degrees of confidence. There is certainly sufficient evidence of biochemical disturbances in manic–depressive psychosis and schizophrenia to sustain the optimism of those who believe that a somatic pathology will eventually be found. But it remains problematical to what extent any biochemical lesion is primary or secondary. It could be the consequence rather than the cause of the psychological symptoms, and even if it is the cause of the symptoms, it may have been precipitated by psychological stresses and continue to be influenced by psychological factors. In other words, there is likely to be a complex interaction of psychological and biochemical factors responsible for the onset of mental disorders and their subsequent course. The 'functional psychoses' would then fulfil the usually accepted criteria of psychosomatic disorders, illnesses with demonstrable somatic pathology in which psychological factors often play a significant part in causation.

The field is still wide open for theories of causation of the common psychiatric disorders. Theories differ in their conceptual framework and may be expressed in the language of neurophysiology, cybernetics, psychology or sociology. Semantic difficulties tend to exaggerate the divergencies between various theories. The main differences lie in the relative emphasis given to hereditary and environmental factors, biological and cultural factors, and physical and psychosocial factors. It is important to bear in mind that these are not either/or categories so much as opposite ends of a continuum. All theories postulate the interaction of multiple variables rather than confining themselves to single pathogenic events such as cerebral anoxia at birth, 'maternal deprivation', or 'social isolation'. All would admit a parallelism between neurophysiological and psychological events, but they might attempt to distinguish between abnormal behaviour arising primarily from abnormal brain function and abnormal behaviour resulting primarily as a response to environmental stress.

Psychodynamic theories

This term usually refers to classical Freudian theory and subsequent theories derived from it which claim that behaviour is determined by the equilibrium achieved between the dynamic forces acting on the individual. Behaviour often appears incomprehensible to the subject or observer because he is not usually conscious of all the motives and conflicts influencing him.

Freud considered that behaviour was chiefly determined by unconscious instinctual drives, whose expression could be partially influenced by the nature of the environment and 'morality'. He postulated a tripartite division of the psychical apparatus into *id*, *ego* and *superego*, with unconscious biological instincts, chiefly sexual and aggressive (*Eros* and *Thanatos*), located in the id. The superego, formed by the introjection of the values and standards of parents, teachers and cultural traditions during early childhood, corresponds roughly to 'conscience'. The ego holds a central position, influenced not only by the id and superego but also by its knowledge of the external environment from sense perception and previous experience. In its attempt to maintain some sort of balance between the demands of the id, superego and reality, the ego is guided by the principles of self-preservation and the avoidance of pain. Threats to its safety and calm may arise from the external environment, ungratified instinctual demands, or the dictates of the superego, and are signalled by anxiety. The ego can react to dangers from the environment (external danger) by consciously determined action such as flight. It reacts to internal dangers (from the id and superego) by employing unconscious defence mechanisms such as repression, reaction formation and regression. These may be relatively successful in removing the threats from consciousness, but at the cost of the resulting neurotic symptoms or character disturbance. Anxiety occupies a central position in the genesis of neurosis, as a signal of danger, which is followed by the blocking of an instinctual drive when its gratification would seem dangerous or impossible, either because of the external environment or because of the superego's disapproval. Situations in which this occur include the threatened loss of a loved person and the threat of punishment (separation, anxiety and castration anxiety). Freud placed greatest emphasis on the sexual drive in the formation of character and behaviour, but it is essential to remember that 'sexual' included any activity which caused bodily pleasure. Adult personality and neurosis depend chiefly on the way the immature ego coped with the oral, anal and phallic stages of the infantile sexual drive. This complex development is biologically determined by the prolonged period of childhood in humans, in which the first love relationship is of necessity incestuous, complete gratification impossible, and the Oedipal conflict arises. It is in infancy that ego development may be impaired or fixated at a particular level and the pattern of defence mechanisms determined. An infantile neurosis is inevitable because of the Oedipal conflict, but need not become manifest in adult life. However, all adult psychoneurosis is the result of either arrested development or the reactivation of the infantile neurosis by the mechanism of regression in response to stress.

It follows from Freudian theory that behaviour is largely unconsciously determined. The instinctual drives, defence mechanisms and part of the superego are not usually accessible to direct observation. They may be inferred indirectly from the content of dreams, slips of the tongue, free association, neurotic symptoms and psychoses. In psychoanalytical theory normal and abnormal behaviour are two ends of a continuum. The type of any mental disorder is determined by the degree of development of the ego and the defence mechanisms employed to maintain an equilibrium between instincts, reality and superego (Freud, 1940; Fenichel, 1946).

Subsequent modifications of psychoanalytical theory have been centred on the origin of aggression, the relative importance of aggressive and sexual drives in the determination of behaviour, the universality of the developmental stages of these drives, the origin of social drives, the extent to which behaviour and personality are influenced by cultural factors, and the degree to which behaviour is determined by the structure of the ego rather than instinctual drives. Present trends have been towards the integration of knowledge from a variety of interrelated disciplines, including the direct observation of child and animal behaviour, the learning theories of experimental psychology and the findings of anthropology and sociology, as well as further psychoanalytical investigations. As a result of this, a more composite picture of the development of personality and patterns of behaviour has emerged, and there is a more flexible approach to the assessment of their determinants.

Alexander and the neo-Freudians, such as Fromm, Horney and Sullivan have placed less emphasis on the paramount influence of the sexual instinct on behaviour. The neo-Freudians stress the influence of social and cultural factors in the development of personality and do not consider all social behaviour to originate from the primary biological drives. The current life situation is given more attention and mental disorder is not always thought to be completely determined by childhood experience. In respect of the more 'orthodox' psychoanalytical developments, the trend towards ego psychology and the analysis of the ego, already evident in both Freud's own later writings and the work of Anna Freud, has continued. Hartmann (1964) has described the development of the ego and its adaptive role in mediating between unconscious instinctual drives and conscious motivation based on environmental factors. Rapaport (1960) stressed the ability of the ego to modify and delay both instinctual demands and the effects of the environment. The concept of ego autonomy allows for the possibility that not all behaviour need be motivated by unconscious conflicts. Holt (1967), reviewing this concept and the problem of free will, draws on the experimental evidence of sensory deprivation and suggests that psychoanalytic theory should be re-formulated in neuropsychological language. Erikson (1965) has described the stages of social development which parallel the psychosexual stages of development.

Introduction

Kardiner *et al.* (1959) also emphasize the role of the ego and the importance of the environment and social learning in the determination of behaviour of the growing child. These new theoretical trends have acted as a counterbalance to the idea that all behaviour is determined by conflict created by the primary drives. It has also allowed a fruitful communication to develop between psychoanalytic theory, ethology and sociology. On the other hand, Melanie Klein has extended psychoanalytical investigation into very early childhood and has stressed the importance of innate aggression in the infant–mother relationship and the inevitable conflict which must arise from this, however good the environment.

Learning theories

There have been vigorous attempts during the last decade to apply knowledge derived from experimental psychology to the problem of psychiatric disorder. The experimental studies of Pavlov, Watson, Skinner, Hull, Spence and others have been used to construct learning principles which could explain the development of human behaviour and indicate methods for its modification. Some of these principles are described in detail in subsequent chapters, but a few general comments are made here. Learning theories, in common with others, accept that both genetic and environmental factors are important in determining abnormal behaviour and that mental disorder is the result of the interaction between a more or less predisposed individual and his changing environment. It is therefore appropriate to consider the extent to which psychiatric symptoms are a form of learned behaviour. According to Eysenck, the susceptibility to neurosis is determined by the personality dimension of *neuroticism*. This is the degree of emotional lability determined by the reactivity of the automatic nervous system. In contrast to this personality dimension, the neurotic symptom is a pattern of abnormal behaviour acquired in a specific learning situation. Any past experiences may have influenced personality development and symptom formation.

Obviously, there are many similarities between psychodynamic and learning theories of behaviour, but at this stage we wish to emphasize some of the differences. Learning theories do not postulate the universal existence of specific intrapsychic conflicts such as the Oedipus complex or the inevitability of infantile neurosis, and they do not consider that the form of neurosis is necessarily determined during childhood.

Treatment

It is customary to describe the treatments employed in psychiatry under three headings, physical, psychological and social. A combination of methods is frequent, and, because many are empirical or symptomatic, there is not necessarily a close correspondence between the theoretical formulation and therapeutic methods selected by the individual psychiatrist. The desire to alleviate suffering is stronger than the wish to be restricted to therapeutic certainty or the rigour of scientific discipline.

Physical treatment

Disorders associated with known organic pathology may respond to specific treatment such as penicillin for cerebral syphilis or surgical excision of a cerebral tumour.

Electroconvulsive therapy (ECT) is an empirical method of treatment used chiefly in severe depressive states, and is often dramatically effective. It may be curative in the depressive psychoses, or alleviate depressive symptoms associated with other disorders such as schizophrenia or obsessional states.

Anti-depressant drugs (not to be confused with euphoriants such as amphetamine and cocaine) can be effective in those types of disorders which respond to ECT, but are usually slower in producing their therapeutic effect.

'Minor tranquillizer' drugs are used in the control of anxiety and agitation. In general they are more effective in acute states of recent onset than in more chronic conditions.

'Major tranquillizers' are not only effective in the control of agitation and excitement, but often have a more broad effect in controlling the disordered thinking, delusions and hallucinations of the psychoses. They are usually employed as the first line of treatment in acute schizophrenia and mania.

Introduction

Leucotomy can relieve severe states of anxiety and tension, and reduce the intensity of manic-depressive psychosis. With skilled surgical technique and careful selection of patients it is possible to obtain good therapeutic results with little or no change in personality or intelligence. It is usually employed in intractable conditions causing prolonged, severe mental suffering and disability in which chronic tension is the central feature.

Social treatment

This includes all measures directed towards providing the social milieu most likely to be free of pathogenic influences and most conducive to the patient's recovery and maintenance of health. Although attempts at environmental manipulation involve a prior assessment of possible pathogenic influences in it, it need not indicate that social factors were of primary importance in aetiology. Help and advice with regard to housing, occupation, family and recreations may be given. The social milieu of the hospital, the 'therapeutic community', 'community care' and the decision between in-patient or out-patient treatment, are all aspects of the attempt to make the maximum usage of beneficial social influences on the patient.

Psychological treatment

This includes all types of psychotherapy from simple reassurance to Freudian psychoanalysis and behaviour therapy. In practice, the treatment a particular patient receives is determined not only by the type of disorder, but also by the theoretical orientation and personality of the psychiatrist and the availability of particular types of treatment.

The various psychotherapies differ in their techniques and therapeutic goals as well as theoretical formulations. Although they all rely on verbal communication, treatment may be carried out individually, or with families or in groups. Frequency and duration of therapies vary greatly. Without too much abuse to the actual range of treatments, it is possible to describe a continuum from supportive psychotherapy to insight therapy, in which there is a rough correlation between the duration of treatment, the extent of the therapeutic goal, the amount of exploration of unconscious material and the concentration on childhood patterns of behaviour in addition to the current life situation.

Freudian psychoanalysis and some of its modifications represent the most ambitious and intensive form of insight therapy, consisting of one-hour sessions four to six times a week for several years. They aim to give insight into the unconscious motivation of behaviour and to allow the development of a healthy character structure. Symptom removal is not necessarily the primary objective but this may occur coincidentally with the attainment of insight and the construction of a healthier personality.

Its chief method is *free association* in which the patient is asked to say everything that comes into his mind without any effort at selection or suppression. The exploration and interpretation of the material of free association and dreams enable some of the important unconscious motivations of the patient to be recognized and experienced. In addition, the ways in which he relates to others and the defence mechanisms he employs are identified by observation of the transference reaction and resistances which emerge during therapy. At the same time as the patient is acquiring insight he has the opportunity of unlearning his neurotic patterns of behaviour by 'working through' and acquiring more healthy modes of relating to others through his experience of a therapeutic relationship with the analyst.

Psychoanalysis can be available to only very few patients because of the amount of skilled manpower involved. For this reason, if for no other, there has been a continuous search for shorter methods of treatment which would still incorporate its therapeutic principles.

Analytically oriented psychotherapy may have the same ambitious goals as psychoanalysis, but treatment can be on the basis of hourly interviews one to three times a week for a much shorter period than full analysis. This is achieved by the therapist playing a more active role in both manipulating the transference and directing the content of the treatment session to those areas which are thought to be the most significant. There is still some free association and exploration of dream material and interpretation of unconscious mechanisms, but there may also be more focus on current problems.

Sullivan's method of therapy may be taken as an example of the neo-Freudian approach. According to Sullivan, the quality of inter-personal relationships, rather than intrapsychic conflicts, are the chief determinants of emotional health. Freedom from tension and anxiety depends on the satisfaction of biological drives and the security en-gendered by social approval. Satisfaction and security can be obtained only by interaction with other people, and patterns of relationship are usually firmly established during childhood. In treatment, the therapist can directly observe the way in which the patient relates to him, and can explore the patient's previous modes of interaction with others. As a result of this the patient may develop an understanding of the unsatisfactory pattern of his interpersonal relationships and learn to modify them so that they may become more emotionally rewarding to him.

In less intensive forms of insight psychotherapy, the emphasis is given to the strengthening of existing healthy personality traits and the modification of maladaptive responses rather than a more radical alteration of personality. Interpretation may be limited to the more conscious conflicts, and attention is focused on current difficulties as much as or more than on childhood experiences. The psychobiological method of Adolf Meyer and Rogers' client-centred therapy fall within this category. In Rogers' client-centred therapy the therapist is active but non-directive. The aim of treatment is to allow the patient to resolve his own difficulties by the use of the healthy part of his per-sonality. The therapist reflects the feelings and clarifies the conflicts as they are presented by the patient, so that he may gradually gain more insight and the capacity to improve his patterns of behaviour. The focus is therefore on the present life situation. There is no interpreta-tion of transference and free association is not employed.

Rogers emphasizes three attitudes that the therapist must adopt in order to create the therapeutic climate in which the patient can improve his own functioning. The therapist must allow himself to be his real self rather than adopting a role, he must show complete acceptance of the patient, and he must have an empathic understanding of the patient. Such a genuinely experienced relationship constitutes the 'necessary and sufficient conditions of therapeutic effectiveness'.

Rational psychotherapy is a directive form of treatment whose aim is the replacement of particular symptoms by a more satisfactory pattern of behaviour. Some explanation of the origin of the symptom may be given together with direct guidance in the development of the new behaviour.

Supportive psychotherapies do not aim specifically either to give insight or to alter personality. Their goal is to remove or alleviate current symptoms as quickly as possible and the techniques employed include the ventilation of problems, reassurance, suggestion, persuasion and direct guidance. These methods are similar to those employed by friends and relatives, but they may be based on a surer foundation as a result of more skilled assessment and the doctor may have the advantage of the status invested in him by the patient.

Psychoanalytical and psychodynamic theory has always encountered a barrage of criticism. Most people now recognize the brilliant insights of Freud and the importance of unconscious motivation, childhood experience and psychosexual development in fashioning adult behaviour. But psychoanalytical theory has been attacked on the grounds that it is not a scientific theory because it does not lead to testable hypotheses capable of refutation (Nagel, 1959; Popper, 1963). Some psychoanalysts accept this criticism but maintain that psycho-analytic theory is a semantic rather than a causal theory and that it provides the patient with a biological theory of the meaning of his experience and behaviour (Rycroft, 1966). The therapeutic efficacy of psychotherapy has been challenged (Eysenck, 1960b) and there is now a large literature on this topic (see Bergin, 1967; Kellner, 1967; Malan *et al.*, 1968; Strupp and Bergin, 1969). The importance of 'non-specific' variables such as suggestion and patients' expectancies in any form of psychiatric treatment has received increasing attention (Frank, 1961, 1968). Freud (1937) discussed the efficacy of analysis in terms of the limiting factors of the intensity of traumas, the strength of the instincts and the strength of the ego. He stressed the limitations of psychoanalysis both in terms of the types of disorder which could be treated and the extent of the therapeutic change which could be expected.

The problem of the range of applicability and therapeutic change in relation to the 'natural course' of psychiatric disorders is discussed in chapter 5. It has been possible to relate certain psychotherapeutic processes to the outcome of treatment but a large number of variables are involved. Patients often improve without specific psychiatric treatment and some patients are made worse by treatment (Bergin, 1967). The most striking feature is that some psychiatric disorders are very persistent and remain uninfluenced by treatment. When neurotic symptoms persist in spite of insight into their assumed cause, it is suggested that the insight is intellectual rather than emotional. But 'emotional insight' is not always a sufficient cause of improvement (Storr, 1966). Furthermore, patients may improve either without gaining emotional insight or after an abreaction involving a fictitious reconstruction of past experience (Sargant, 1957). The apparent great resistance to modification by verbal means of some psychiatric disorders has been accounted for in a variety of ways. Both psychodynamic and learning theories emphasize the adaptiveness as well as maladaptiveness of symptoms (the *neurotic paradox*). Many theorists also distinguish between cognitive and emotional learning processes. There are some similarities between the primary and secondary processes postulated by Freud and the first and second signalling systems of Pavlov. Language and cognition may be expected to influence behaviour established with verbal awareness, whereas emotional and behavioural responses acquired without cognitive awareness may require 'corrective emotional experiences' or other actual behavioural responses in order to modify them.

Behaviour therapy

Behaviour therapy aims to modify current symptoms and focuses attention on their behavioural manifestations in terms of observable responses. The techniques used are based on a variety of learning principles. Although behaviour therapists adopt a developmental approach to the genesis of symptoms, they do not think that it is always necessary to unravel their origin and subsequent development.

There are considerable differences in the treatment techniques employed in behaviour and psychodynamic therapies. The principles and experimental findings from which behaviour therapies have been derived have led to such procedures as the systematic construction of hierarchies of anxiety-provoking situations, carefully graded training programmes and specific schedules of positive or negative reinforcement. These techniques are used rarely, if at all, in psychodynamic therapies.

There are also features common to both methods of treatment. History-taking, the expectancy of the patient, the relationship between patient and therapist, suggestion, persuasion, encouragement (whether or not verbalized) are shared by most methods of treatment.

If at this stage we try to underline their difference without caricaturing them, we would emphasize the predominantly verbal method of psychodynamic treatments, their aim to give understanding of present behaviour and their specific exploration of attitudes and feelings. Behaviour treatments make more use of non-verbal methods and have as their primary aim the modification of behaviour rather than an understanding of it.

Chapter 2

Principles of Conditioning and Learning

Although the potential range of behaviour of any organism is genetically determined, environmental factors play an important part in determining actual behaviour. Learning refers to any relatively permanent change in behaviour which occurs as a result of practice or experience. Not all behaviour is learned; changes due to physiological processes such as growth or ageing, and short-lived effects such as fatigue and adaptation, are excluded.

Learning covers a wide range of behaviour, from simple conditioned reflexes to complex conceptual learning. The term 'conditioning', as used in present-day psychology, is applied to two relatively simple experimental procedures, known as classical and instrumental (operant) conditioning. A vast amount of psychological research has been concerned with the investigation of the processes underlying conditioning. In our present state of knowledge there is a considerable area of agreement concerning the experimental findings in conditioning, but considerable controversy among theorists in the concepts and hypotheses formulated to explain the data.

A comprehensive review of conditioning and learning would be impossible in a single chapter, and we shall attempt to describe only some of the main theories and findings in this field which seem most relevant to the aetiology and treatment of psychiatric disorders. For a full review of this subject, the reader is referred to Kimble (1961), from which much of the material in this chapter is drawn. It is worth emphasizing at this stage that much of the experimental work has been concerned with simple laboratory learning by animals, which may or may not have much relevance to the usually more complex learning situations of human beings outside the laboratory. This is not the place to argue the advantages of the analytic or the synthetic approach.

Both have their merits and demerits. But as long as one remains wary of over-generalizing from a simple situation to a more complex one merely by analogy, it seems worthwhile to analyse the processes underlying simple learning, firstly because it is easier to analyse simple than complex behaviour, and secondly, because complex behaviour may in fact be due to chains of simple behaviour or at least involve similar processes. At present, however, the relationship between simple animal learning and human conceptual learning remains uncertain and generates highly emotionally-charged controversy.

Classical conditioning

This procedure was first introduced and systematically studied by Pavlov (1927). A hungry dog usually salivates at the taste of food. This is an unconditioned reflex. When the dog salivates at the sound of a bell preceding the presentation of food, a conditioned reflex has been established. The dog has acquired the ability to make a particular response to a previously neutral stimulus. In a typical experimental conditioning procedure, a bell is sounded immediately before food is presented to a harnessed hungry dog. After several trials in which the bell is paired with food, the dog salivates as soon as the bell is sounded. The bell has become a conditioned stimulus (CS) which evokes the conditioned response (CR) of salivation. Before the experiment, only the food, the unconditioned stimulus (UCS), evoked salivation, the unconditioned response (UCR).

Pavlov's classical conditioning procedure with dogs has been successfully extended to many other species, from flatworms to human beings from infancy onwards. A wide variety of responses have been conditioned, including autonomic responses such as sweating, heart rate, gastrointestinal secretions, nausea, vomiting, and skeletal responses such as tendon jerks and limb withdrawal.

Certain empirical findings in classical conditioning have been established. Some of these also seem to apply to other forms of learning.

(a) *Acquisition*. The strength of the conditioned response increases in an asymptotic curve as the number of trials in which the UCS and CS are paired increases.

(*b*) *Extinction*. As the number of trials in which the CS is presented without the UCS is increased, the conditioned response diminishes and eventually disappears.

(*c*) *Spontaneous recovery*. If there is a period of rest after extinction, the CR tends to re-emerge. This tendency is more marked after continuous than distributed practice of the response during extinction.

(*d*) *Generalization*. This is the tendency to respond to similar stimuli in the same way. The dog who has been conditioned to salivate to the sound of a certain frequency will also salivate in response to sounds of higher and lower frequencies. The strength of the CR varies with the similarity of the stimulus to the original CS. The dimensions of stimulus generalization are determined by the symbolic meaning as well as the physical properties of the stimulus. A good example of this is provided by studies of semantic generalization. Razran (1939) established conditioned psychogalvanic skin responses (PGR), to verbal stimuli. A subject conditioned to respond to the word SURF showed a greater conditioned response to the word WAVE than to the word SERF, thus showing that meaning was more important than physical similarity in determining stimulus generalization. A recent review of semantic generalization is provided by Feather (1965).

Response generalization is the counterpart of stimulus generalization. If a particular CR is no longer possible, the organism reacts to the CS with a different but similar response. For example, a dog will lift another foot to the CS if the foot which was usually lifted is tied down.

(*e*) *Discrimination*. It is possible to condition the organism to discriminate between similar but non-identical stimuli which had previously evoked an identical response, by extinguishing one of the conditioned responses. A dog conditioned to salivate to a circle and an ellipse can be trained to differentiate between them if one of the stimuli (e.g. the ellipse) is repeatedly presented without the UCS (food), until it no longer salivates at the sight of an ellipse.

(*f*) *Higher order conditioning*. A well-established CR can be conditioned to a new CS by pairing it with the original CS without the UCS. A dog conditioned to salivate to the sound of a buzzer can then be conditioned to salivate at the sight of a black triangle if this is paired with the buzzer. In other words, the buzzer, the original CS, is now acting as an UCS. The triangle is a second-order CS. Pavlov was unable to attain more than third-order conditioning with dogs, because the original CR extinguishes before fourth-order conditioning can occur.

One can speculate about the adaptive value to the organism of discrimination, generalization and higher order conditioning. History never repeats itself exactly, and we are never faced with an exactly identical environment. Without generalization and higher order conditioning, conditioned responses would never be evoked outside the laboratory. Without discrimination, adaptive modification of the conditioned response to a changing environment would not occur.

Instrumental conditioning

The great value of studying classical conditioning lies in the relative simplicity of the learning situation and the possibility it affords of determining the variables and processes which govern it. However, it is obvious that classical conditioning is an example of a very restricted and artificial form of learning. This has led some psychologists, notably Thorndike (1911) and Skinner (1938), to introduce less restricted experimental conditions which allowed the study of more complex forms of learning. They differ from the Pavlovian procedure in that the animals' own behaviour determines whether the UCS is presented. The response to be conditioned must occur before the UCS and is instrumental in producing the UCS. The animal is therefore exerting some active control over the environment rather than passively reacting to it. Instrumental conditioning has been employed for centuries by animal trainers, parents and teachers. It has been studied in the laboratory during the last seventy years. The most commonly used experimental procedures are as follows:

Reward training. Here the performance of some response leads to a goal object for which the animal is motivated (Kimble, 1961). Typical experimental conditions include cats in puzzle boxes or rats in T-mazes who are rewarded with food if they escape from the box or run the maze correctly. Another procedure uses rats or pigeons in a Skinner box, which is a small compartment containing a movable lever. Depression of the lever releases a pellet of food into the box. An animal placed in the box will sooner or later press the lever and obtain food.

Gradually it learns to press the lever to obtain food. The stimulus of being placed in the Skinner box usually leads to a period of apparently random trial-and-error behaviour until the lever is pressed (CR), which is instrumental in the production of food, the UCS. Training a dog to shake hands is an example of the practical application of this procedure.

Escape training. In this procedure the subject must make a particular response in order to terminate a painful stimulus (UCS). In a typical experiment, an animal is placed on an electrified grid and is given a mild shock without warning. The shock activates a pain–fear response, involving cerebral, autonomic and neuroendocrine mechanisms, together with various aversive skeletal responses. Following the performance of a particular skeletal response, the experimenter terminates the shock. After a few such trials, the animal learns to make this response (escape response) as soon as it receives the shock.

Avoidance training. Escape training becomes avoidance training if the experimenter presents a signal (CS) before the painful stimulus and allows the animal to avoid the shock by responding promptly to the signal. In this training the animal learns both how to escape the shock (an instrumental conditioned response) and a classically conditioned fear response to the signal. With further trials the escape response occurs as soon as the signal is presented, and therefore becomes an avoidance response. This technique has been subjected to detailed investigation by Solomon and his associates (Solomon and Wynne, 1953, 1954; Turner and Solomon, 1962).

Avoidance responses differ from other instrumental responses in that they have been shown to persist through hundreds of trials in which no shock has been administered after the warning signal. More recently, Turner and Solomon (1962) have extended this technique to human subjects and have demonstrated that it is possible to set up stable avoidance responses to a neutral CS which are quite resistant to extinction.

Schedules of reinforcement. Skinner (1938, 1953) has used a variant of instrumental conditioning, operant conditioning, to study the quantitative relationships underlying this process. It has been possible to extend the investigation of operant conditioning from laboratory experiments with animals to human behaviour in a less restricted environment. Instead of a series of discrete trials as used in most reward training, Skinnerian methods utilize a free-responding situation. When the organism makes an appropriate response it is immediately free to make the same response again. Under these conditions, the progress of learning can be measured in terms of rate of responding – the number of responses per unit of time.

Since reinforcement of operant behaviour (the provision of rewards) is not necessarily regular and continuous in real life, Skinnerians have investigated the effect of various schedules of intermittent reinforcement as opposed to continuous reinforcement on operant conditioning. Intermittent reinforcement is given either on a time-interval basis or after a certain number of correct responses. In addition, the schedule may be fixed or variable. Each of these four types of schedule has a characteristic effect upon the rate of responding and extinction (Ferster and Skinner, 1957).

The importance of single reinforcement was brought out in two experimental procedures which have come to prominence in Skinner's work – *superstitious behaviour* and *shaping*.

Superstitious behaviour. A response which has been conditioned because of the 'accidental' relationship between it and subsequent reinforcement is termed superstitious (Skinner, 1948). For example, if a pigeon is given food every fifteen seconds – a fixed-interval schedule (FI) – whatever behaviour the pigeon is engaged in when the food is given, such as standing in one corner, becomes conditioned and tends to become a prominent part of its behavioural repertoire. This occurs even though the food is given according to a time schedule unrelated to the bird's behaviour. The use of the word 'superstitious' in such a context immediately invites a comparison with some human behaviour. Perhaps the rituals of the gambler before throwing the dice or the bowler before his run up share the same basis as the pigeon's behaviour.

Shaping. Because organisms tend to repeat the responses which occurred at the time of reinforcement, it has been possible to produce progressively more complex forms of behaviour in gradual stages from a preceding simpler form. Suppose one wishes to teach a pigeon to peck at a small disc on the wall. Reinforcement is first given when the bird moves towards the disc and remains there. The next reinforcement is given when the bird raises its head towards the disc. Each subsequent reinforcement is given as the bird progresses further towards the target and pecks it. This type of operant conditioning or shaping has successfully produced quite complex behaviour patterns.

Comparison of classical and operant conditioning

These two types of conditioning have been defined operationally. The main differences are:

1. In classical conditioning the UCS is given irrespective of the organism's own behaviour. In instrumental conditioning, the organism's own behaviour determines whether or not the UCS will be presented.

2. In classical conditioning the time interval between the CS and the UCS is rigidly fixed. In instrumental conditioning the time interval depends on the organism's own behaviour.

3. In classical conditioning the CR and UCR are similar but not identical. In instrumental conditioning such similarity is the exception rather than the rule.

4. Responses which can be classically conditioned tend to be either those mediated by the autonomic nervous system – such as salivation or heart rate – or relatively involuntary reflexes – such as eye-blinking or tendon jerks. Instrumental responses that can be conditioned tend to be movements which are more obviously under voluntary control and mediated by the central nervous system. In fact it seems that responses which can be conditioned by one method cannot be conditioned by the other, although there may be a superficial resemblance between certain classical and instrumental responses. The theoretical implications of this difference are considered in the discussion of two-factor theory (pp. 41–3).

On the other hand the two types of procedure have many features in common in that they are influenced in a similar fashion by many of the experimental variables studied. The only important exception is that partial reinforcement (reinforcement of only a proportion of the trials) is more detrimental to the establishment of classical than to that of instrumental conditioning. However, despite this exception, it appears that similar principles underlie both conditioning procedures. The crucial experiments of comparing the conditioning of the same response by the two methods is not possible because in practice it is impossible to perform a purely classical or instrumental procedure.

Main variables affecting learning

Learning was defined as any relatively permanent change in behaviour resulting from practice. Change in behaviour refers to observable performance and is assessed by measures such as amplitude, latency, rate of response and probability of occurrence. However, learning really implies the acquisition of the potential to perform certain acts, rather than their actual performance. It is therefore a hypothetical construct which can only be inferred from observed change in performance, which is the translation of learning into actual behaviour. Most learning theories emphasize this difference between learning and performance. It is very difficult to investigate the individual contributions of learning and performance variables because of the difficulty in separating them. However, there is evidence to suggest that motivation, intensity of the conditioned stimulus, amount of reinforcement, and distributed as opposed to massed practice influence performance.

With regard to practice, as the number of conditioning trials is increased, the strength of the CR is increased. However, there is some ambiguity in the meaning of the term 'practice'. Learning can take place as a result of reading instructions on a map without overt rehearsal of the response to be performed. Classical conditioning can occur when the usual external stimulus is replaced by direct stimulation of the central nervous system and even when the overt motor response is prevented. 'Practice' therefore seems to be mediated by some critical neurophysiological process in the central nervous system.

Reinforcement

A further qualification has to be added to the term 'practice' in our operational definition of learning, in order to distinguish between learning and extinction. Unreinforced practice leads to extinction, whereas reinforced practice strengthens learning. Reinforcement is defined empirically as any event which, when employed appropriately, increases the probability of a particular response recurring in a similar situation. There is some confusion in terminology, but Skinner refers to reinforcing events as positive or negative, according to whether their presentation or removal acts as reinforcement. Food is a positive reinforcer, pain a negative one. Negative reinforcement differs from punishment which is defined by Skinner as the removal of a positive reinforcer or the presentation of a negative one. Some writers, however, call punishment negative reinforcement. Punishment does not have the same effect as absence of reinforcement, but leads to temporary suppression rather than extinction.

Some quantitative relationships between reinforcement and performance have been established as a result of experimental research. Performance appears to increase as a negatively accelerated function as the amount of positive or negative reinforcement increases. In classical conditioning, optimal results are obtained when the CS is presented 0·5 seconds before the UCS. Longer or shorter intervals produce weaker conditioning, and if the UCS is presented before the CS (backward conditioning), almost no learning takes place. Intermittent reinforcement leads to greater resistance to extinction than continuous reinforcement. Instrumental responses which are spatially or temporally closer to reinforcement are learned more quickly than those responses which are more remote. This phenomenon is often referred to as the *gradient of reinforcement*. The degree to which remote reinforcement is effective appears to be a function of the organism's level of development – older children and adults are usually more easily reinforced by a promised or delayed reward than are younger children and animals who require tangible and immediate reward. Allied to the gradient of reinforcement is Mowrer's finding that behaviour followed by a small but immediate reward and a large but delayed punishment tends to be preserved, whereas small but immediate punishment may lead to elimination of behaviour even though a large reinforcement follows later (Mowrer, 1950).

Reinforcement has been defined operationally because of the difficulty in formulating a theoretical definition. This has been criticized on the grounds of circularity, but Skinner points out that a reinforcing stimulus is one which increases the probability of repetition of a behavioural response in the future. This is an empirical definition which avoids circularity so long as reinforcement is not employed as a causal explanation. Meehl (1950) has argued that the definition of reinforcement is not tautological because a reinforcing event identified in one learning situation is likely to have reinforcing properties in quite different learning situations as well. Another criticism levelled against the concept of reinforcement is that it implies that a causal agent follows the event it explains. But this again is based on a mis-understanding of the use of the term and is invalid as long as reinforcement is not used in a causal sense or it is identified by its effect on the probability of future behaviour. To state that reinforcement increases the probability of recurrence of the behaviour which preceded it is analogous to the statement that concussion decreases the probability of recurrence of the behaviour which preceded it (retrograde amnesia). The phenomena of reinforcement and retrograde amnesia present a problem with regard to the neurophysiological processes which mediate them and have given rise to the hypothesis that reinforcement and concussion occur at a time when they can strengthen or disrupt the consolidation of neural pathways activated by preceding behaviour. But this is a problem in physiology and not a problem in logic. It is not yet clear why a reinforcer reinforces, although there are a variety of tentative explanations. Psychological theories range from 'psychic satisfaction' to the 'pleasure principle' of psychoanalysis. Physio logical explanations involve concepts such as drive reduction or homeostasis.

Returning to the empirical description of reinforcers, food, water, sex, and pain are called *primary* reinforcers because they are concerned with basic physiological needs. Many reinforcers, however, are acquired in a similar way to the acquisition of classical conditioned reflexes. In order to establish a *secondary* reinforcer, a neutral stimulus is paired with a primary reinforcer until it acquires the capacity to act as a reinforcer on its own, and is able to retard the extinction of a response or establish the learning of a new response. An example of the rewarding nature of secondary reinforcement is shown by an experiment by Bugelski (1938), with two groups of rats conditioned to press a lever to obtain a pellet of food delivered with a clicking noise in a Skinner box. During extinction trials, the clicking noise was continued for one group and eliminated for the other. The lever-pressing response was extinguished less quickly in the group in which the clicking noise was continued. In other words, the noise acted as a secondary reinforcer in delaying extinction in the absence of primary reinforcement. Similarly, neutral stimuli paired with the presentation of noxious stimuli acquire aversive properties. The conditioned avoidance learning previously described depends on the conditioning of a secondary reinforcer. Another example of new learning established by secondary reinforcement (Miller, 1948) is shown by rats conditioned to escape from a white compartment into a black one after having been given a shock in the white one. After this escape response was well established, the shock was never used again, but the rats continued to escape from the white to the black compartment as soon as they were placed in the white one. The white box had become a conditioned aversive stimulus (secondary negative reinforcer). There is considerable evidence that the variables which influence classical and instrumental conditioning have a similar effect on the establishment of secondary reinforcers.

In addition to their ability to strengthen responses, primary reinforcers have a motivational function. Similarly, secondary reinforcers can acquire motivational properties in the sense of acting as goals which stimulate behaviour. The concept of secondary reinforcement has been used by some learning theorists to account for a variety of experimental findings. For instance, the ability of partial reinforcement to increase the resistance of a response to extinction may be due to the effect of a secondary reinforcer having been established during acquisition which continues to occur in the trials without primary reinforcement.

One of the most important aspects of secondary reinforcement lies in its ability to influence behaviour before and until primary reinforcement occurs. Hull (1952) put forward the concept of 'fractional anticipatory goal responses' to account for the observed sequence of behaviour in complex problem solving in which primary reinforcement is delayed until the final correct response is completed.

The principle of secondary reinforcement and motivation gives some indication of the influence of learning on motivation. Money or tokens have been successfully conditioned as secondary reinforcers with incentive value for chimpanzees. Acquired drives obviously activate much human behaviour which is not directly or immediately related to primary drives such as hunger or sex.

Imitation

Most human learning takes place in a free environment in which language and the observation of other people's behaviour play a prominent role. Bandura has pointed out that the teaching of language or complex skills like driving a car by operant conditioning techniques would be extremely laborious. Furthermore, trial-and-error methods of acquisition of new behaviour patterns would be very hazardous in a natural environment in which an error may prove fatal. In real life, as opposed to the laboratory, social imitation plays an important part, particularly in the acquisition of novel responses. Bandura emphasizes the greater efficacy of imitation over shaping procedures in the acquisition of language. There is good experimental evidence that subjects can acquire a generalized tendency to make imitative responses by operant reinforcement techniques in which the observer is rewarded directly (Baer and Sherman, 1964). Miller and Dollard (1941) demonstrated that both rats and children can be taught to imitate a model in place learning by rewarding them for correct choices. However, Bandura and his associates (Bandura and Walters, 1963; Bandura 1965a and b) have focused attention on vicarious no-trial learning, in which the subject learns new responses as a result of observing the behaviour of others and its reinforcing consequences on them without making any overt response himself or receiving any direct reinforcement. In one experiment children were shown a film in which an adult behaved aggressively in a manner which would be novel to the children. Although the children did not make aggressive responses or receive reward during the time they were watching the film, they displayed the aggressive responses after the film. The performance of imitative behaviour by the subject is influenced by the observed reinforcing consequences of the model's behaviour. There is less imitative behaviour by the observer when the model is punished rather than rewarded. The subject is influenced by 'vicarious reinforcement'.

There is evidence that maladaptive behaviour can be acquired and extinguished by modelling procedures. These topics are discussed in subsequent chapters. With regard to the theoretical basis of imitation, Bandura considers that neither classical nor instrumental conditioning procedures provide a satisfactory paradigm for vicarious no-trial acquisition of novel responses. In common with many learning theorists, he distinguishes between learning and performance, but also maintains that learning is established by contiguity of stimuli arising from the subject's perception of the model and the central responses of imagery and thought which they evoke. These symbolic responses may then serve as discriminative cues which control the subsequent overt performance of the imitative responses.

Theories of learning

In our present state of knowledge it is often impossible to identify the neurophysiological processes which underlie learning and performance. Explanatory theories can be couched in physiological or psychological terms according to the use which we wish to make of them. Physiological theories may be expressed in terms of neurochemical or electrical changes. Differing patterns of EEG activity in classical and instrumental conditioning (Galambos and Sheatz, 1962) suggest that different physiological processes are involved in the two types of conditioning. A brief review of the brain mechanisms involved in learning is provided by Pribram (1961).

Understanding of the physiological processes which mediate behaviour and learning might lead to the development of more efficient physiological methods of facilitating learning. Unfortunately, the complexity of neurophysiology has so far prevented this. This is one reason why psychologists have devoted more time to the elaboration of psychological theories. Eloquent pleas for the integration of physiological and psychological approaches have been made by Hebb (1955) and Razran (1965).

Historically, learning theories have been concerned with two major issues, what is actually learned and whether reinforcement is always necessary. With regard to the first problem there have been two major schools of thought, one (e.g. Guthrie, 1935; Skinner, 1938; Hull, 1943) maintaining that stimulus–response connexions are learned (s–r theory), the other (e.g. Tolman, 1932) that stimulus–stimulus associations are learned (s–s or cognitive theory). It should be remembered, as Pribram (1963) has pointed out, that even the reflex arc proposed by Sherrington to account for spinal reflexes, was only considered to be a 'useful fiction'. Complex human behaviour cannot possibly be accounted for by such a simple process. The latency of the 'response' in much human behaviour indicates that more than a single s–r link is involved. Theoretical constructs and intervening variables are required to explain this, whether of the form of anticipatory goal responses (Hull), mediating processes (Osgood), or cognitive links. MacCorquodale and Meehl (1954) have given a formal definition of Tolman's construct of 'expectancy' and show how similar it is to Hull's construct of 'habit'. The points at issue in this controversy really centre round the meaning of the terms 'stimulus' and 'response'. Some learning can take place without obvious overt responses. The organism seems to learn to perceive its environment in a new way. Examples of this have been provided by perceptual learning, sensory preconditioning (Brogden, 1939), learning without responding (under curare paralysis), place learning and latent learning. But it is impossible to exclude the possibility that some covert 'response' is not being made in these situations. Thoughts and feelings are often experienced, and some peripheral responses of very small amplitude such as mouthing words or changes in tone of muscles which would mediate the overt response may occur in addition to central nervous activity. But as Hebb (1958) has forcefully commented, to class visual perception as a 'response' in the same category as a skeletal movement broadens the concept beyond its usually accepted meaning. Some types of learning therefore seem to be accounted for more readily in terms of s–s theory than s–r theory. As both theories have to account for the same experimental findings, they can only afford to differ in their theoretical constructs.

With regard to the second major issue in learning theory, whether reinforcement is necessary for learning, some s–r theorists have maintained that reinforcement is always required (e.g. Hull, 1943). However, it can be difficult to identify the reinforcing agent in some learning situations, even when the concept of reinforcement is enlarged to include primary rewards of exploration and arousal (Hebb, 1955; Berlyne, 1960) and secondary reinforcement. It appears that there is no simple mechanism underlying the process of reinforcement. Drive reduction, the presentation or removal of a stimulus, or the elicitation of a response may all have reinforcing properties. At present there is no single theory which accounts for all the empirical data of reinforcement. In consequence of this, the search for all-embracing theories has given way to the more modest employment of restricted theory to account for particular phenomena of learning. Of the multi-process theories, the most popular is the two-factor theory (e.g. Mowrer, 1947; Skinner, 1938; Schlosberg, 1937) which maintains that classical (respondent) conditioning occurs without reinforcement and that instrumental (operant) conditioning requires reinforcement. One potent influence on the development of two-factor theory was the difficulty encountered in explaining the phenomena of avoidance learning. The avoidance response is evoked by a painless warning stimulus and prevents the organism from experiencing the noxious stimulus, thus eliminating the basis of reinforcement in terms of drive reduction (removal of pain). Drive theorists found it difficult to account for the maintenance of avoidance behaviour in the absence of this reinforcement. Two-factor theory maintains that in early trials the warning signal (CS) acquires the ability to evoke fear (CR) as a result of contiguity and classical conditioning. Once the warning signal itself evokes fear, the avoidance response reduces the fear and is therefore reinforced by this drive reduction (instrumental learning). Conditioned fear is often referred to as anxiety or conditioned avoidance drive (CAD).

It has still been found difficult to account for the very great resistance to extinction of conditioned avoidance responses. Solomon and Wynne (1954) have put forward two principles, anxiety conservation and partial irreversibility of anxiety, in an attempt to explain this phenomenon. According to the first principle, the avoidance response has a shorter latency than the conditioned anxiety response, so that avoidance action occurs before the conditioned anxiety is fully developed. In this situation little or no anxiety reduction is experienced by the organism, and the avoidance response is no longer reinforced. The reduction in reinforcement leads to an increase in the latency of the avoidance response until the conditioned anxiety is fully developed again and the avoidance response is reinforced. As a result of this there is a waxing and waning of the anxiety response and rapid extinction by massed practice of unreinforced trials is prevented. In order to account for the absence of even slow extinction, the principle of partial irreversibility of anxiety has been invoked. According to this, severe trauma can cause irreversible physical changes in the organism which prevent the complete extinction of the response. The evidence in support of these two principles is far from clear-cut, but it remains a well-established fact that ordinary extinction procedures are very often ineffective in eliminating instrumental avoidance responses.

Another aspect of the two-factor theory is the proposal that the organism's responses can be divided into two basic types, according to the learning process by which they can be modified. Skinner (1938) makes the distinction between elicited and emitted behaviour. Responses evoked by known stimuli are called elicited responses – for example, salivation at the sight of food – and are dependent upon respondent (classical) conditioning. Responses which appear independently of specific identifiable stimuli are called emitted or operant responses, to indicate that they 'operate on the environment to generate consequences'. Operant responses are subject to the rules of operant (instrumental) conditioning. They include those parts of the organism's behavioural repertoire mediated by the central nervous system such as speech and skeletal muscular movements. Mowrer (1950) has developed this dual nature of learning very clearly, distinguishing between the classical conditioning of predominantly involuntary emotional, visceral and vascular responses, mediated by the autonomic nervous system, which act as anticipatory states increasing drive, and instrumental conditioning, which establishes voluntary responses which are mediated by the central nervous system and are problem-solving, pleasure-giving and drive-reducing. More recently, however, experiments which purport to demonstrate the operant conditioning of autonomic responses have been published (Fowler and Kimmel, 1962; Frazier, 1966; Rice, 1966; Dicara and Miller, 1968). There is considerable controversy concerning the significance of these findings. In a recent review, Katkin and Murray (1968) draw a distinction between *conditioning* autonomic responses as opposed to *controlling* autonomic responses. They point out that autonomic responses may mistakenly be assumed to have been established by an operant conditioning procedure when in fact they may be unconditioned or classically conditioned responses to external or internal stimuli occurring during the operant conditioning procedure. This accentuates the point made by Kimble that it is not possible in practice to prevent the occurrence of classical conditioning during an instrumental conditioning procedure.

Extinction

So far we have been concerned chiefly with conditioning processes – the acquisition of responses – and have not considered the processes involved in the extinction of behaviour. The basic experimental procedure for obtaining extinction is non-reinforced practice. If the CS for example the bell – is presented without UCS (food), the CR (salivation) gradually decreases and finally fails to occur. This decrement cannot be regarded simply as a passive decay, since conditioned responses display only a very limited tendency to diminish solely with the passage of time. Evidently the elimination of conditioned responses, sometimes in a brief session of unreinforced practice, depends on some active process. A number of different opinions exist about this.

Two concepts, both borrowed from reflex physiology, predominated in the earlier theories of extinction. The first was the concept of *inhibition* which postulated that any non-reinforced response generated an inhibitory tendency opposing the reproduction of that response, and that the inhibitory tendency increased with the number of non-reinforced trials, but decreased with the passage of time. This theory of inhibition is consistent with the phenomenon of spontaneous recovery, and the greater effectiveness of massed than distributed practice in producing extinction. However, some other findings, particularly the greater resistance to extinction of responses established with intermittent rather than continuous reinforcement, are difficult to account for in terms of inhibition theory.

The second concept was that of *interference*, which postulated that any new response interfered with the evocation of the previously learned response and so supplanted it. However, the origin of the new response and its reinforcement is not accounted for. Furthermore, this view assumed that extinction was due to the conditioning of a new incompatible response. Yet there is evidence to suggest that conditioning and extinction are functionally different. For example, massed practice and depressant drugs tend to delay learning but accelerate extinction, whereas distributed practice and stimulant drugs accelerate learning but delay extinction.

In an attempt to overcome the inadequacies of both inhibition and interference theories, Hull (1943) developed a two-factor theory combining elements of both. He suggested that both reinforced and non-reinforced responses produce a state of reactive inhibition, having the properties of a primary drive, similar to fatigue. Reactive inhibition will lead to the cessation of the response and a rest period which allows the reactive inhibition to decay. The reduction of reactive inhibition reinforces the resting response and leads to conditioned inhibition which interferes with the previous conditioned response, causing its permanent extinction. Hull's two-factor theory is more satisfactory than either inhibition or interference theory but still fails to explain some of the experimental findings in extinction (Gleitman, Nachmias and Neisser, 1954), such as the extinction of fairly effortless responses like the PGR or extinction obtained without responding (under curare). Conditioned inhibition also fails to explain the differences in resistance to extinction of partially and continuously reinforced responses.

An additional hypothesis put forward by many theorists is that of *generalization decrement*. In experimental conditioning, the response is influenced by many or all of the stimuli present in the learning situation. It has been shown that changes in these 'environmental' stimuli as well as any change in the 'main' CS will lead to a decrement in the strength of the CR. As a consequence of this, the rate of extinction will be influenced by the degree of similarity between the environmental setting of the acquisition and extinction trials. Alteration of the time interval between extinction trials leads to more rapid extinction than that obtained when the inter-trial interval is the same in extinction and acquisition trials. The hypothesis of generalization decrement is also of some value in explaining the resistance to extinction of partially reinforced responses. Partial, as opposed to continuous reinforcement, would lessen the differences between acquisition and extinction trials, and therefore diminish generalization decrement in the extinction trials.

Another effect of partial reinforcement (if positive) is the omission of positive reinforcement (frustration) experienced in the unrewarded trials. There is some evidence that this type of frustration is a drive which can energize behaviour and facilitate interference responses. Frustration would therefore be expected to delay acquisition in early trials, but strengthen the response in later trials and increase its resistance to extinction. This theory would account for the more rapid extinction of continuously reinforced responses, in which the organism is subjected to the interfering effect of frustration for the first time during extinction.

Expectancy theorists also postulate that extinction results from interference responses. However, these new responses are thought to result from the change in the expectancy of the organism as it realizes that reinforcement is no longer forthcoming. It follows from this that the rate of extinction will depend on the speed with which the organism perceives the difference between the acquisition and extinction situations. Partial and variable schedules of reinforcement during acquisition trials resemble extinction trials more than continuous and fixed schedules do, and would therefore make discrimination between them more difficult. Experimental findings show that these schedules do in fact lead to greater resistance to extinction. Expectancy theory embodies some aspects of generalization decrement and interference theory.

Our present understanding of the phenomenon of extinction has reached a similar stage to our understanding of learning and reinforcement. Most of the empirical observations are not in dispute, but it is necessary to employ a number of different hypotheses to explain them. However, we should not be too ashamed at having to use multifactor theories, for as yet the evidence suggests that extinction, like learning and reinforcement, is not a single phenomenon, but includes a variety of different processes.

Principles of Conditioning and Learning

Summary

In this chapter we have attempted to review briefly some aspects of learning. We have relied heavily on laboratory experiments investigating simple forms of learning in animals. A number of generalizations concerning relationships between the variables involved, which would command agreement among most psychologists, have been established.

It is obvious that most human learning and behaviour appears vastly different to the seemingly trivial conditioning procedures studied in laboratory animals. Human learning generally takes place in a free environment and often in a social setting. Language plays a very important role and complex conceptual processes are involved. The early theories of behaviourism could not satisfactorily account for such learning in terms of classical and instrumental conditioning alone. Neo-behaviourism has extended its theoretical range to overcome some of these deficiencies with concepts such as expectancy, fractional anticipatory responses, gradients of reinforcement and chaining of responses. More emphasis is placed on organismic variables and individual variation. The gap in the behaviouristic account of social conduct has been recognized and there is good evidence that social imitation is an important primary mode of learning.

At the beginning of this chapter we adopted a cautionary attitude to the relevance of animal conditioning procedures to human learning. Some theorists maintain that the laws of conditioning apply to all learning, or that conditioning is actually the basic unit of all learning. Complexity is thought to result from the simultaneous and cumulative effects of many simple events. Internal (covert) behaviour such as thoughts and feelings are assumed to be subject to the same basic laws of learning. At the other extreme are those who hold the view that no permutation of conditioning processes could account for the complete range of human learning and that advocacy of this view involves unwarranted extrapolations from animal laboratory experiments and tenuous analogies.

At the present time there is no satisfactory, single, all-embracing theory to account for the phenomena of human learning. It is not yet possible to decide between the two opposing views of the importance of conditioning. The principles of conditioning have not yet been fully elucidated, and even less is known about the manner in which simple conditioned reflexes combine and function together in human behaviour. However, there is no evidence to suggest that conditioning is irrelevant in human learning and it may prove fruitful to continue to explore the possibility of accounting for complex learning in terms of simple units.

Chapter 3

Learning Theory Formulations of Psychiatric Disorder

The basic approach of the behaviourist towards psychiatric disorders is to assume, in the absence of contrary evidence, that learning processes are important in their development and maintenance. This is not to deny that genetic, maturational, or organic disease processes may play a part; but the behaviourist emphasizes the role of learning and tries to see how far psychiatric disorders can be explained in terms of learned maladaptive patterns of behaviour. As already discussed in chapter 1, a majority of psychiatrists and behaviourists do not subscribe to an organic concept of neurosis and personality disorder, but consider them as multifactorially determined patterns of behaviour differing quantitatively rather than qualitatively from normal behaviour.

Although all behaviour theorists agree on the importance of learning processes in the formation of abnormal behaviour, they vary in their theoretical formulations because of the absence of any single, unified learning theory. Obviously the problems concerning the nature and necessity of reinforcement, or cognitive and s–r theories, are relevant to the acquisition of abnormal as well as normal behaviour. Some behaviour therapists adopt Hull's learning theory, some adopt a two-factor theory, while others attempt to eschew theory and employ Skinner's system. An additional difficulty in elaborating an aetiological theory of psychiatric disorder is the paucity of critical experimental evidence concerning the establishment of abnormal human behaviour, so that reliance has to be placed on clinical evidence, analogue studies and animal experiments.

The majority of learning theorists (e.g. Hull, Mowrer, Dollard, Miller, Wolpe, Eysenck) postulate that anxiety plays a central role in the neurotic disorders, agreeing with Freudian theory in this respect.

However, learning theorists conceptualize 'neurotic anxiety' as a conditioned emotional response (CER) which may have subjective, autonomic and skeletal motor components, established by the process of classical conditioning in which a previously neutral external or internal stimulus was paired with an aversive stimulus. As a result of this conditioning and subsequent stimulus generalization and higher-order conditioning, anxiety may be evoked by many stimuli which have no primary aversive property. The conditioned anxiety also has the properties of an acquired drive, sometimes referred to as conditioned avoidance drive (CAD), and can therefore activate and reinforce an instrumental escape or avoidance response. In other words, the acquisition of 'neurotic anxiety' is thought to follow the traumatic avoidance learning paradigm discussed in the previous chapter (p. 31), consisting of a classically conditioned emotional response followed by an instrumental avoidance response and anxiety reduction.

Let us consider how well this model can account for neurotic disorders. The classic experiment of Watson and Rayner (1920) demonstrated that it is possible to condition anxiety in such a way. They were able to establish an anxiety response to a white rat in an eleven-month-old boy (Albert) who had previously shown no fear of it, by making a loud noise by striking a steel bar (UCS) whenever Albert approached the rat. After several presentations, a conditioned anxiety response was well established, had generalized to other furry animals and objects, and persisted for over a month. If the fear and avoidance of furry animals persisted it could be considered a maladaptive response because in this situation rats are neither dangerous nor usually paired with a loud noise. In this sense it is analogous to a 'neurotic fear'. This experiment therefore provides some evidence that neurotic fear can develop as a result of classical conditioning in which emotional reactions evoked by aversive stimuli become conditioned to previously neutral stimuli. Krasnogorski (1925, 1933) reported the classical conditioning of anxiety reactions in children by using strong electric shock or difficult discriminations.

In Watson's experiment, several presentations of the aversive stimulus were given. However, a single presentation of an intense aversive stimulus can lead to stable emotional responses (Hudson, 1950; Campbell *et al.*, 1964). Campbell describes the establishment of stable

CER in human subjects following single-trial learning with succinyl-choline-induced respiratory paralysis as the unconditioned aversive stimulus. Obviously this is an unusual and frightening experience which is unlikely to be a common cause of naturally occurring human neurosis, but may be relevant to the development of acute traumatic neuroses such as those which occur in battle or following disasters, in which a large number of exposed subjects develop psychological reactions (e.g. Grinker and Spiegel, 1945; Tyhurst, 1951; Popovic and Petrovic, 1964). However, there is also experimental evidence that repeated exposure to mild aversive stimuli can lead to persisted CERS (Pavlov, 1927; Liddell, 1944; Wolpe, 1952). This may be more analogous to the natural development of human neurosis. There is some evidence that repeated exposure to mild aversive stimuli may lead to CERS which are of greater intensity than the original UCR; Wolpe (1958) put forward a highly speculative model to account for this. In brief, he suggested that the anxiety evoked by the CS in the previous trial is added to the anxiety evoked by the CS and UCS in the subsequent trial. Eysenck (1968a) has put forward a theory of incubation to account for this phenomenon. He suggests that the fear response evoked by a conditioned aversive stimulus may be a painful event which is self-reinforcing, so that whether an increment or extinction of response occurs on repeated exposure to an unreinforced conditioned aversive stimulus will depend upon the balance between incubation and extinction existing at the time. Incubation is more likely to occur when the UCR is strong. It could account for the clinical finding that a phobia may increase in severity in the course of time without re-exposure to the original traumatic situation (such as a road accident) having taken place.

The first major difficulty encountered in proposing classical conditioning as the basis for neurotic anxiety reactions is the problem of their persistence. If they depend on classical conditioning, extinction should take place after re-exposure to the CS unless it is paired with the UCS. Clinical evidence does indeed suggest that extinction of CERS frequently occurs. Taylor (1966) points out that only a minority of subjects develop persistent anxiety or other neurotic reactions following an acute trauma. The majority of people involved in road accidents, for instance, do not develop persistent travel phobias. Eysenck and

Rachman (1965) maintain that the majority of conditioned fears are extinguished and therefore subject to 'spontaneous recovery' (in the sense of clinical cure). Certainly, surveys of fears in children and adults suggest there is an association between the incidence of particular fears and age (Jersild and Holmes, 1935; MacFarlane *et al.*, 1954). Obviously maturational processes may be more relevant than reinforcement history in determining the occurence and duration of childrens' fears. But even in adults, surveys of 'normal people' show that 'irrational fears' are not uncommon. However, the irrational fears of normal people often differ from the phobias of patients seeking treatment in that they are less intense and do not sufficiently restrict their activities to interfere with ordinary life.

The evidence suggests that the majority of anxiety responses to specific stimuli are extinguished or at least do not become persistent and disabling. Yet there is good experimental evidence that stable CERS can be acquired easily and CARS are extremely resistant to extinction (Solomon and Wynne, 1954). Both in humans (Campbell *et al.*, 1964) and in dogs (Napalkov, 1963) repeated exposure to the CS alone can lead to strengthening of the CER. Eysenck (1968a) has accounted for this in terms of his theory of incubation. The stability of traumatic avoidance learning has been accounted for by Solomon and Wynne in terms of anxiety conservation and partial irreversibility of anxiety. In effect, anxiety conservation implies that the avoidance response effectively prevents the subject from experiencing sufficient anxiety in the presence of the phobic stimulus for extinction to take place. The patient, by avoiding crowded lifts, gives himself no chance of discovering that crowded lifts are not really dangerous. When no effective CAR is available because the subject is confined, the CER is likely to be more intense and more resistant to extinction. In general, there is a reciprocal relationship between intensity of the CER and the CAR after the first few trials, so that unavoidable punishment generates more anxiety than avoidable or escapable punishment. Mowrer and Viek (1948) found that rats shocked in an inescapable situation developed more severe disruption of feeding than rats who had received the same amount of shock, but who could escape from it.

As already discussed in chapter 2, there are other theoretical interpretations of traumatic avoidance learning. In the field of animal neuroses, for example, Wolpe (1958) employs the concepts of reinforcement by drive reduction and the slowness of extinction by reactive inhibition to account for the persistence of neurotic anxiety. He argues that the anxiety response is predominantly an autonomic one which generates less reactive inhibition than do skeletal responses, so that extinction by conditioned inhibition will be slow. Secondly, he points out that eventually the anxiety is reduced when the animal is passively removed from the experimental situation and the anxiety reduction reinforces the CER. Wolpe admits that there are objections to this theory. Certainly, much experimental evidence suggests that the onset rather than the offset of the UCS reinforces fear responses, so that drive reduction does not seem to be crucial (Kimble, 1961). On the other hand there is good evidence that confinement in the experimental situation combined with prevention of avoidance does lead to extinction of the fear response (see Lomont, 1965).

It seems, therefore, that traumatic avoidance learning can provide a model for the development of neurotic anxiety reactions which fail to extinguish because of the intensity of the emotional response or avoidance behaviour which prevents re-exposure to the aversive stimulus. A variety of procedures have been used to induce experimental neuroses in animals. In the majority of them, the animals have been confined in the experimental situation and exposed to either noxious stimulation or some sort of conflict situation. Single exposure to intense traumatic stimuli or repeated exposure to milder stimuli has led to persistent CERs and CARs in dogs, cats, sheep and goats (Pavlov, 1927; Liddell, 1944; Wolpe, 1952). Variables affecting the strength and persistence of the 'neurotic' behaviour include the intensity and frequency of noxious stimulation, degree of confinement, possibility of escape or avoidance, drive state and individual differences (hereditary or previous experience). Among the primary aversive stimuli which have been used in the experimental conditioning of emotional and avoidance responses are electric shock, blasts of cold air, loud noise, toy snakes and severed heads. It must be emphasized, however, that stimuli not causing tissue damage and not necessarily causing physical pain may still be aversive. Species differences and degree of maturation are important factors determining which stimuli evoke unconditioned aversive responses.

Learning Theory Formulations of Psychiatric Disorder

There is considerable controversy concerning the importance of conflict as a cause of experimental and human neuroses. Pavlov (1927) induced experimental neuroses in dogs by a variety of procedures such as an increasingly difficult sensory discrimination, prolongation of the interval between CS and UCS, and increasing or altering the aversive stimulus used as a CS for salivation. Liddell (1944) employed difficult discriminations with sheep and goats, while Masserman and Wolpe used an approach–avoidance conflict by pairing food with an aversive stimulus. A number of different theoretical formulations have been suggested to account for these experimental findings. Pavlov postulated the conflict or clash between 'excitatory' and 'inhibitory' cerebral processes resulting from the simultaneous elicitation of positive and negative conditioned responses. Liddell postulates that in his experimental procedures the combination of monotony and persistent vigilance for the animal leads to 'neurotic behaviour'. These are both neurophysiological rather than psychological models. Gantt (1953) elaborated the concept of 'schizokinesis' to describe his experimental finding that dogs continued to exhibit cardiac acceleration responses to CS long after the secretory and motor components of the CR had been extinguished. The amount of cardiac acceleration following a CS for food was greater than that accompanying ordinary muscular exercise and comparable to that associated with strong emotional states. Gantt postulates that there is a cleavage between the cerebral processes mediating autonomic and skeletal responses resulting in a maladaptive persistence of cardiac responses to CS. His suggestion that the neurotic dog 'remembers with his heart' echoes Breuer and Freud's dictum that 'hysterics suffer mainly from reminiscences'. Some caution is required in the interpretation of cardiac responses, because deceleration or acceleration may occur and it is not always easy to predict the direction of the response without detailed knowledge of the experimental situation and previous history of the organism (e.g. Lacey et al., 1963).

There is now a considerable literature on the effects of drugs, electric shock and expectancy on the conditioning of emotional and avoidance responses (e.g. Stephens and Gantt, 1956; Brady, 1957; Bridger and Mandel, 1965; Sachs, 1967). They may enhance emotional and reduce avoidance responses and so induce 'neurotic states' or they may inhibit emotional and facilitate avoidance responses and induce 'fearless' behaviour. The relevance of these findings lies not only in their resemblance to neurotic behaviour and therapeutic activity but also in the fact that conditioning procedures and cognition may also have a similar effect.

Masserman (1964) considers that the motivational conflict between fear and hunger is the crucial factor in the production of experimental neurosis in his investigations. He puts forward experimental evidence obtained with eighty-two cats from which he concluded that neither aversive stimulation alone, spatial constriction, nor mechanical prevention of the feeding response led to persistent neurotic behaviour. Wolpe (1952), however, produced similar patterns of neurotic behaviour with noxious stimulation alone, and argued that conflict is not a necessary condition. It is possible that differences in experimental procedure are responsible for these conflicting results and that Wolpe used stronger aversive stimuli. Although Wolpe maintains that conflict is not a necessary condition for experimental neurosis, he agrees that ambivalent stimulation in which opposing responses tend to be elicited simultaneously in approximately equal measure is a sufficient cause of experimental neurosis. Such a conflict situation is capable of evoking emotional responses and previously established avoidance responses (Fonberg, 1956). Hunt (1961) has suggested operationally that conflict situations may be considered to be aversive stimuli because their onset is punishing and their termination rewarding. It is worth emphasizing that behaviourists, like psychodynamic theorists, accept that conflict can be an important antecedent of emotional and avoidance behaviour. The behaviour of Masserman's cats exposed to an approach–avoidance conflict showed a strong superficial resemblance to some aspects of human neurosis. Generalized anxiety, restlessness, autonomic disturbances, excessive startle responses, increasing anxiety in situations similar to the experimental situation, starving rather than eating whilst in the cage, avoidance and ritualistic behaviour were among the manifestations described. Miller's (1944) analysis of approach–avoidance conflict has been employed by Dollard and Miller (1950) as a model for the learning of human neuroses. They suggest that conflict rather than single drives provide the majority of painful circumstances in the living of our lives and enumerate the frequent occasions in which either difficult discriminations or conflicting drives are likely to arise during the course of childhood development and social training. The reason why conflict or ambivalent stimulation in which noxious stimuli are not involved is aversive or anxiety evoking is not clear. Neurophysiological theories such as the disruptive effect of combined excitatory and inhibitory stimulation require further explanation. Broadhurst (1960) makes use of the Yerkes–Dodson law and suggests that difficult discriminations in the experimental neurosis procedures may lead to levels of drive which are too high for the complexity of the task and so result in disruptive and emotional behavioural responses. Yates (1962) has reviewed the experimental studies of frustration and conflict.

Further evidence of the importance of conflict in the genesis of psychiatric disorder is provided by a study of a psychosomatic disorder in which Sawrey *et al.* (1956) found that the combination of hunger and electric shock in an approach–avoidance conflict led to the development of more stomach ulcers in rats than the effect of hunger or shock alone.

The discussion so far has leaned heavily on the conditioned emotional and avoidance responses produced in animal laboratory experiments in which the behaviour disturbances bear some resemblance to human neurosis. Among the more obvious differences between experimental animal neurosis and human neurotic disorder are the complex conceptual processes involved in human neurosis. Language and imagery can function as response-produced cues which evoke anxiety and avoidance responses. Thinking about or imagining situations which in reality evoke fear is often sufficient to cause subjective anxiety and autonomic responses. Introspection and measurement of autonomic responses confirm that anxiety occurs in association with exposure to verbal instruction or suggestion. Anticipation of electric shock (Bridger and Mandel, 1964) and hypnotic suggestion (Barker, 1965) are examples of this. Language allows semantic and symbolic generalization to occur with the result that conditioned anxiety responses may generalize to a large number of new stimuli. Speech, thought and imagery enable emotional and avoidance responses to occur and recur without any exposure to a conditioned aversive reality situation. Not only does this enormously increase the range of circumstances in which emotional responses can occur, but it may also be responsible for increasing their resistance to extinction. Conditioning and generalization may occur without conscious awareness and there is some evidence that this leads to less adaptive and more persistent emotional responses (Lacey and Smith, 1954). Hefferline (1962) emphasizes the relevance of response-produced cues in human behaviour, pointing out that all organs of the body have sensory receptors. Much human behaviour may become contingent on 'internal' cues, whether thinking or other somatic processes, and it may be difficult to relate these to external environmental stimuli. Eriksen (1958), however, while accepting that conditioning can occur without verbal awareness, remains cautious about its interpretation in terms of unconscious mechanisms. Another method in which emotional and avoidance responses may be acquired without direct experience of traumatic or conflicting stimuli is by observation. Imitation, as emphasized by Bandura, is a potent method of human learning, and fears may develop as a result of this. Jones (1924a) described a child who developed an anxiety response to rabbits after observing another child in the same play-pen show fear of a rabbit. A number of experimental studies have illustrated that conditioned fears can be acquired vicariously by observation of a model showing fear when exposed to the object (Berger, 1962; Murphy *et al.*, 1955; Miller *et al.*, 1962, 1963; Bandura, 1965b; Bandura and Rosenthal, 1966). The significant correlations found by May (1950) and Hagman (1932) in the incidence of fears in children and their siblings and mothers suggests that at least there is an opportunity for their being acquired by imitation. The explanatory hypotheses put forward to account for neurosis in terms of conditioned fear still leave many aspects unexplained. If it is accepted that the conditioned emotional and avoidance responses resulting from strong aversive, multiple mild aversive or ambivalent stimulation are analogous to human neurosis, there is still no single agreed theoretical explanation of their origin or persistence. Related to this is the difficulty of accounting for the fact that phobic disorders represent a small minority of the neurotic disorders seen in psychiatric practice. The answer that conditioned anxiety responses may often be associated with a variety of behavioural responses including successful avoidance and resultant diminution of the emotional response (symptoms and defence mechanisms in psychodynamic terminology) presents the problem of elucidating the variables which determine the choice of the neurotic behavioural response.

The occasional reference to individual differences influencing behavioural responses in experimental neurosis procedures suggests that these may be of importance. There is ample evidence that there are significant differences in physiological and psychological responses to the environment. Personality variables, whether genetically determined or shaped by previous experience, are considered to be important by the majority of theorists. Pavlov (1927) postulated four major personality types based on the Hippocratic temperaments – sanguine, choleric, phlegmatic and melancholic – to account for the different responses of his dogs. Eysenck (1957), also following Hippocrates, postulated that the non-cognitive aspects of personality can be subsumed under two dimensions, neuroticism and extraversion. Neuroticism is considered to be an innate predisposition determining the reactivity and lability of the autonomic nervous system. Neurotic disorders are more common in those with high neuroticism because their more frequent and intense emotional responses afford more opportunities for the conditioning of fear or instigation of impulsive action. The dimension of introversion–extraversion in Eysenck's system is characterized by the ease of conditioning which is mediated by the inferred cerebral inhibitory and excitatory balance. Introverts condition easily because of the preponderance of cerebral excitation, whereas extraverts condition less easily because of the preponderance of cerebral inhibition. There is some evidence that the speed of classical conditioning of eyeblink is related to personality traits such as anxiety (Spence, 1964) and introversion (Eysenck, 1957; Franks, 1960). Eysenck suggests that introverts with high neuroticism scores are likely to develop dysthymic disorders (anxiety, phobias, depression, obsessions), while extraverts with high neuroticism scores are liable to develop hysterical or psychopathic disorders. Eysenck has accumulated much evidence in support of his personality theory. However, a certain number of studies do not support or even contradict his theory. Davidson *et al.* (1964, 1966) and Becker and Matteson (1961) have not found the expected correlation between GSR conditioning and introversion. Bunt and Barendregt (1961) failed to find a general factor of conditioning. Eysenck, however, considers that these experimental findings do not conclusively invalidate the theory which may, tentatively at least, be accepted as tenable (Eysenck, 1965; Eysenck and Rachman, 1965). More recent studies (Kelly and Martin, 1969; Martin, Marks and Gelder, 1969) have failed to show the expected correlations between neuroticism and autonomic reactivity, or between introversion and condition ability. Eysenck's theory of personality structure has served as a stimulus for research and leads to testable hypotheses. That some modifications are likely to be required to account for more complex findings does not detract from its heuristic value. From the clinical viewpoint, it seems likely that the type and degree of autonomic reactivity would be important factors in both psychosomatic disorders (e.g. Lacey and Smith, 1954) and anxiety and phobic neuroses. There is evidence that patients with chronic anxiety states and agoraphobia show higher levels of arousal and slower habituation as measured by PGR (Lader *et al.*, 1967) and a higher forearm blood flow (Kelly and Walter, 1968) than patients with isolated phobias or normal controls. It has been suggested by some authors (e.g. Lader and Mathews, 1968; Snaith, 1968) that the high level of arousal of patients with anxiety states and agoraphobia is more important than specific traumatic conditioning events in the maintenance of their disorder, in contra-distinction to subjects with specific phobias in which traumatic conditioning is likely to be the most important factor.

It is therefore possible in theory to account for some of the diversity of behaviour disturbances and their occurrence in only a proportion of a population who appear to have been exposed to not grossly dissimilar environmental circumstances in terms of learning influenced by personality variables. Our analysis of the learning situation so far might be relevant for acute traumatic neuroses and relatively isolated phobic disorders. But the majority of patients seen in clinical practice do not appear to fit easily into either of these categories. In many specific phobias it is not possible to trace their historical origin and there is no reliable method of establishing the validity of the historical reconstruction. The patient may have no conscious recollection of the origin and no awareness of important stimuli which currently evoke anxiety.

Factors which would be expected to be important in determining the choice of phobic objects include the frequency of exposure and intensity of the primary aversive stimuli, drive level, personality variables, age and the nature of the environmental stimuli at the time of conditioning. It seems probable that the more distinctive stimuli and those which have previously elicited anxiety will become conditioned aversive stimuli. Other people may become conditioned aversive stimuli, such as the parent or teacher who punishes or rejects the child, particularly if this is done frequently. In such a case generalization to other adults or all authority figures could result in severe disturbances in interpersonal relationships. When either covert responses such as wishes, thoughts, fantasies, or interoceptive responses have become conditioned aversive stimuli, there may be no obvious external stimulus or awareness on the patient's part of the anxiety evoking cue. If conditioned, covert, response-evoked aversive stimuli can be avoided in the same way as external stimuli, 'repression' can be conceptualized as the conditioned avoidance of ideational stimuli. 'Free floating' anxiety could result from extensive stimulus generalization and higher-order conditioning in any of the above situations. The strength and frequency of aversive conditioning and the speed of the subject's conditioning will be the determining variables. In addition, a CS which evokes fear may also increase the strength of unconditioned responses to other aversive stimuli (Brown *et al.*, 1951). Moreover, some components of a conditioned emotional response may themselves be response-produced primary aversive stimuli. For example, autonomic and skeletal responses may cause visceral pain, bronchospasm, nausea or vomiting which in turn evoke anxiety. This describes in terms of peripheral events a process similar to the self-reverberating circuit or functional autonomy usually formulated in terms of neurophysiological circuits or habit strength. Some emotional responses are associated with physiological processes which are longer acting and less flexible than other responses in that they may continue long after the original stimulus situation. For instance, changes in cortisol secretion rate and hypertrophy of the adrenal glands may be persistent or progressive and lead to pathological changes or death despite removal of the organism from the apparent instigating stimulus situation. Animals have died after being placed in cages in which other animals were already established (Clarke, 1953; Barnett, 1958). Another example is provided in the experiments of Brady *et al.* (1958) by the 'executive' monkeys who died after being subjected to traumatic avoidance conditioning. Apart from these autonomic and endocrine responses which may themselves have aversive or learned drive properties, continuous or 'free floating' anxiety may be maintained by recurrent exposure to aversive stimuli in the external or internal environment. Wolpe (1958) suggests that anxiety may become conditioned to 'pervasive aspects of experience' such as awareness of space, time, and one's own body. The conditioned response may include rumination over unpleasant or frightening thoughts and images which increase anxiety, or there may be an ongoing conflict situation such as an undesired marriage which will cause continuing anxiety.

There is little theoretical difficulty in explaining the occurrence of generalized and persistent anxiety, but many of the theories proposed are at a level of generality which precludes them from having much predictive value or being capable of experimental refutation. But if we accept that neurotic disorders often result from anxiety reactions to noxious or conflicting stimuli, we still have to consider how the choice of symptom is determined. In the model of traumatic avoidance learning, the resulting behaviour may be any combination of emotional or instrumental avoidance responses. Anxiety and its autonomic manifestations may appear together with a wide range of motor responses. 'Freezing', withdrawal, motor excitement, stereotypy of movement and reappearance of previous avoidance responses have been observed in animal experimental neuroses and human traumatic neuroses.

In order to understand the development and content of symptoms it is important to identify the type of stress which induced them and the individual's response to the stress. Early childhood experience provides many opportunities for aversive conditioning to take place. But it can be difficult to identify the origin of symptoms with any degree of certainty. Freud pointed out that the psychoanalytical approach, like any other historical approach, succeeds in making a reconstruction in retrospect only. Prospective studies are needed to demonstrate the relationship between childhood training and adult personality and behaviour. There is no shortage of speculation. The quality of the mother–child relationship has been emphasized by many. Bowlby (1951) developed the concept of maternal deprivation in infancy as a cause of the subsequent affectionless delinquent personality. The absence of good mothering was thought to prevent the child from experiencing and therefore learning to love and trust his mother, and this would generalize to prevent the child from making positive relationships. Much work has been conducted on maternal deprivation since Bowlby's original study and it is now recognized that this does not necessarily lead to personality or neurotic disorder and that when it does its effect is not specific, because a variety of psychiatric disturbances may result (W.H.O., 1962). A large literature has amassed on the effects of childhood bereavement with conflicting results (see, for example, reviews by Dennehy, 1966; Granville-Grossman, 1968). However, there is some evidence that behaviour disorder, suicide and depressive disorders are associated with childhood bereavement. Learning theorists would predict that lack of or unsatisfactory childhood training could lead to the development of psychiatric disorder. This could be permanent if there were critical periods of learning in human development similar to those found in other species. The well-known work of Harlow (1963) on monkeys reared apart from their mothers and peers illustrates the potentially devastating effect of grossly adverse early experience. Isolation of infant monkeys for eighteen months leads to long-lasting impairment of heterosexual and social behaviour. This degree of interference with normal childhood is exceptionally rare and can hardly be a common cause of human neurosis. But lesser degrees of deprivation, rejection or inconsistency of parental training are common and might be expected to lead to psychiatric disorder. Here again, the methodological problems involved in testing such hypotheses are enormous and no simple relationships between types of upbringing and psychiatric disturbance has been established.

Hewitt and Jenkins (1946) described three patterns of abnormal behaviour in children attending the Michigan Child Guidance Clinic which correlated with distinctive types of parental upbringing. Unsocialized delinquency was associated with overt parental rejection, whereas 'socialized delinquency' was associated with neglect rather than rejection. Excessive parental repression led to neurotic overinhibited behaviour in the child. Clinical impressions have given some support to such a relationship although a recent validation study on a sample of approved school boys failed to identify the parental upbringing patterns (Field, 1967).

The aetiology of obsessional neurosis remains obscure. Obsessional and compulsive symptoms can occur in association with organic brain disease, depressive illnesses or schizophrenia and their course is then usually related to the associated psychiatric disorder. In man, obsessional symptoms are defined by their experiential characteristics of subjective compulsion and wish to resist them (Lewis, 1957), with the result that many repetitive acts, rituals and impulses do not fall within this category. Whether or not this is a distinction with causal implications remains to be established, but, in the meantime, caution is required in assessing the relevance of repetitive or ritualistic behaviour of animals to human obsessional symptoms.

A variety of methods have been employed to induce stereotypy or fixated responses in animals. Maier (1949, 1956) found that a majority of rats develop fixated responses, either positional or symbolic, when presented with the combination of an insoluble discrimination problem and noxious stimulation. The fixated response may persist even when the problem is made soluble, no noxious stimulus is presented, and the correct response has been learned. Special methods were required to eliminate the fixated responses. The persistence and resistance to extinction of these is reminiscent of traumatic avoidance learning. The use of noxious stimulation in these experiments may therefore be a crucial factor in the persistence of the responses. In other words, any motor component of an active avoidance response emitted frequently because of the stimulus or drive conditions of the organism might appear to be a repetitive or fixated response and the parameters influencing it will be the same as those influencing avoidance conditioning. The strength of the aversive or conflict stimuli, previous reinforcement history, drive level and individual differences will be important determinants. Aversive stimuli will increase the strength of instrumental avoidance responses previously established by negative reinforcement and, if mild, may act as a discriminatory cue to strengthen instrumental responses established by reward (Solomon, 1967).

The experimental work discussed so far has come within the category of avoidance learning and anxiety reduction. Another example of experimentally induced repetitive motor responses is the 'superstitious' behaviour established in pigeons by operant conditioning. In this case, coincidental motor responses occurring at the time of reinforcement become conditioned and the pigeon may develop seemingly senseless 'ritualistic' behaviour. It is possible that this is analogous to human rituals, such as mannerisms or repetitive ideas and thoughts, which are performed because they have been associated with positive reinforcement previously. In birds, reinforcement of consummatory behaviour too early in the response chain may lead to seemingly senseless or maladaptive repetitive motor responses (Hinde, 1960). Another method of inducing stereotyped behaviour has been described by Berkson (1967). Chimpanzees reared in isolation displayed body rocking movements similar to those found in mentally subnormal children. This stereotyped behaviour was more frequent when the level of anxiety was high and when the animals were in a restricted and bare environment. It seems that repetitive and apparently maladaptive motor responses may therefore arise as part of a repertoire of avoidance or approach responses.

In man, the ideational component of obsessive–compulsive behaviour is very prominent. Often the compulsive thoughts or rituals appear to be avoidance responses in so far as their performance reduces anxiety while attempts to resist them lead to an increase in anxiety. For example, a patient may wash his hands ten times in order to eliminate the idea and accompanying anxiety that his hands are contaminated and will lead to his infecting anyone who touches anything his hand has touched. However, the handwashing ritual is secondary to the idea of being contaminated (Lewis, 1957) and it is only these secondary symptoms which appear to be anxiety-reducing responses. The origin of the obsessional idea of contamination (the primary symptom) still has to be accounted for. Some obsessional fears, for instance a fear of being killed, could be the ideational component of a previously conditioned emotional response, but there is often no apparent fear stimulus preceding the obsessional fear. Interoceptive or internal stimuli of which the patient is unaware may be functioning as conditioned fear stimuli. Whether or not this is so (there is some controversy concerning the role of unconscious conditioned stimulus generalization), the prominence of the ideational component, its repetitiveness and persistence, remain the important features to be accounted for. In adults, the neurosis usually occurs in patients who have an obsessional personality with orderliness, conscientiousness, high ethical standards and indecisiveness (Kretschmer, 1934; Pollit, 1960; Ingram, 1961; Rosenberg, 1967). The patients' compulsive rituals bear some resemblance to the magical and superstitious thinking of young children and the ceremonial rituals accompanying taboos (Freud, 1918; Flugel, 1945). If these observations are considered together, one could speculate that compulsive behaviour is the learned avoidance response to the type of conflict situations met in childhood in which anxiety is engendered by the presence of any drive whose reduction is difficult because of its anticipated punishing and therefore anxiety-evoking consequences. The choice of 'magical', 'superstitious' or ritualistic avoidance behaviour may be determined by developmental factors, for it is part of the behaviour repertoire of children and primitive societies when confronted with approach–avoidance conflicts.

Metzner (1963) considers that psychoanalytical theory locates a source of conflict in childhood which enables some sense to be made of the content of symptoms but fails to give a satisfactory account of the precipitating and maintaining conditions. Those compulsive symptoms which appear to be evoked by definable environmental aversive stimuli can be subsumed under the category of previously learned traumatic avoidance responses. But Metzner admits that this is not a satisfactory explanation of 'fixated' and apparently 'senseless' ritualistic acts in response to anxiety evoked by 'internal' ideas and impulses. These cases may be similar to the animal analogue experiments in which either randomly inflicted punishment or punishment of an avoidance response leads to its fixation. Metzner suggests that the child who has learned to believe that 'dirty' thoughts can be washed away like physical dirt may respond with handwashing when he becomes anxious because of sexual impulses. The handwashing will only temporarily reduce anxiety and the sexual impulse will continue to recur. The avoidance response is unsuccessful and the handwashing becomes fixated and develops into crippling ritualistic behaviour. By chance, handwashing may occur at a time when anxiety lessens, so that intermittent reinforcement will increase its resistance to extinction.

Some hysterical reactions can be considered to follow the traumatic avoidance-learning paradigm. Hysterical symptoms are often precipitated by obvious traumatic situations, in war neuroses (Grinker and Spiegel, 1945) or natural disasters. They may occur simultaneously with acute anxiety or panic or be accompanied by a characteristic calm – *belle indifférence*. In the latter case it may be functioning as an effective anxiety avoidance response, a view which receives some support from evidence that the removal of hysterical symptoms can lead to the emergence of anxiety (e.g. Freud, 1909; Dollard and Miller, 1950; Brady and Lind, 1961). When anxiety and hysterical symptoms co-exist, presumably their avoidance function is only partially successful. Wolpe (1958) suggests that hysterical symptoms occur as conditioned responses to stress in the same way as anxiety symptoms, but that in some people or some particular situations the hysterical responses are prepotent. Eysenck (1957) considers that hysterical symptoms will occur in lieu of anxiety symptoms in response to stress more frequently in extravert than introvert subjects because the more rapid conditioned inhibition of extraverts facilitates 'blocking' and other inactive responses such as paralyses and mitigates against the establishment of more active avoidance responses. Clinical evidence suggests that hysteria is a threshold phenomenon in that increasing the stress will increase the incidence of hysterical reactions. Hysterical symptoms are more frequent in childhood and in states of impaired consciousness and brain damage. In this respect the incidence of hysteria may parallel some types of suggestibility. It seems likely that hysterical symptoms may be both an unlearned and a conditioned response to traumatic situations. Personality differences, degree of maturation and level of consciousness may be relevant variables. Some 'global' hysterical symptoms such as amnesia and twilight states may be undifferentiated and unconditioned responses to intense fear. But why particular hysterical symptoms occur is not at all clear. Sometimes they appear to imitate symptoms that have been experienced previously by the patient during the course of an organic illness or observed in other people. Hysterical aphonia, for example, may occur after an attack of laryngitis or after seeing someone with a hoarse voice due to carcinoma of the larynx. Psychoanalytical theory emphasizes the symbolic meaning of the symptom in relation to the repressed instinctual impulse.

Learning theory can account for the maintenance of a specific hysterical symptom in terms of operant conditioning. The hysterical symptom (operant response) emitted at the onset of the hysterical reaction may be influenced by the presence of discriminative stimuli and the previous reinforcement history of the patient, but its subsequent course and shaping will be contingent upon its reinforcement by a positive reinforcer (e.g. sickness benefit) or by escape from a negative reinforcer (e.g. mother-in-law). Operant reinforcement is the equivalent of the 'secondary gain' of the hysterical symptom in psychoanalytical terminology. The 'primary gain' is translatable into learning terms as its function as an avoidance response which reduces anxiety evoked by a stimulus of which the patient is not fully aware. Explanations of hysterical reactions in terms of role playing and communications can be subsumed under the operant conditioning paradigm.

Psychosomatic diseases (defined as diseases with demonstrable somatic pathology in which psychological factors can play an important role in causation or maintenance) can be incorporated within a learning framework as long as genetic and constitutional factors are included. The major premise is that the well-recognized but usually reversible autonomic and neuroendocrine components of anxiety and other emotional responses may lead to permanent tissue changes under certain circumstances. In other words the raised blood pressure accompanying anxiety may become fixed, prolonged mucosal engorgement of stomach and bowel combined with increased cortisol secretion may lead to haemorrhage or chronic ulceration. If this is the case, the same learning situations which lead to persistent anxiety or avoidance responses could also lead to psychosomatic disorders. Intense, recurrent or sustained exposure to aversive stimuli or conflict would be one of the necessary conditions for the acquisition of a psychosomatic illness by conditioning. But one of the disputed areas in psychosomatics is the problem of 'organ choice'. Why duodenal ulcer rather than hypertension? Why ulcerative colitis rather than an anxiety neurosis? Learning theorists must again invoke individual differences resulting from the combination of heredity, constitution and previous learning. Individual differences in patterns of autonomic reactivity to stress stimuli are apparent at the age of six and remain stable through the course of time. There are also consistent differences in the individual subject's autonomic responses to different types of stress (Lacey and Lacey, 1958; Lacey *et al.*, 1963). The demonstration of individual variation in patterns and intensity of autonomic responses to stressful stimuli could account satisfactorily for the differential incidence of psychosomatic disease and there is in fact some evidence of a relationship between the patient's pattern of autonomic reactivity and his psychosomatic symptoms (Malmo and Shagass, 1949; Malmo *et al.*, 1950).

Support for the hypothesis that psychosomatic disease may result from conditioned emotional responses has come from animal experiments. Traumatic avoidance conditioning led to peptic ulceration in the experimental 'executive' monkey but not the control monkeys (Brady *et al.*, 1958). Sawrey *et al.* (1956) induced peptic ulcers in rats submitted to an approach–avoidance conflict. Although not usually classified as a psychosomatic disease, failure to thrive and early death has been described by Liddell (1960) in lambs and kids subjected to a one-hour stressful conditioning schedule while separated from their mothers. In these experiments the relative contributions of the conditioning procedure and the separation from mother remain to be clarified.

There is both experimental and clinical evidence that some psychosomatic disorders are due to the additive effects of allergy and emotion. Asthma and hay fever attacks have been precipitated by the combination of pollen sprayed into the room and anxiety evoked during an interview but not by either alone. Asthmatic attacks have been conditioned to a variety of stimuli including photographs of a horse or the patient's mother (Dekker and Groen, 1956; Metcalfe, 1956). This indicates how somatic disorders may come to be evoked by 'psychogenic' or previously neutral stimuli as a result of classical conditioning, stimulus generalization and higher-order conditioning. Operant conditioning may also play a part in psychosomatic disorders. Turnbull (1962) has discussed the aetiology of asthma and indicated the manner in which classical and operant conditioning may be involved.

Certain types of alcoholism and drug addiction can also be conceptualized as learned avoidance behaviour mediated by anxiety and maintained by anxiety reduction. Alcoholism has been experimentally induced in animal experiments (e.g. Conger, 1956) and learning theory formulations of addiction have been constructed in terms of anxiety reduction, with reinforcement provided by the combination of pharmacological action, conditioned reinforcement, and the social milieu in which some addicts live. Wikler (1968) has put forward an account of relapse in terms of conditioning.

Our discussion so far has been based largely on disorders with relatively discrete patterns of behaviour which can be encompassed within the framework of anxiety and avoidance responses, derived from possibly analogous animal experimental neurosis. But human behaviour disorder is usually complex, occurs in a social setting, is accompanied by a prominent ideational component, and does not always appear to be mediated by anxiety or its avoidance. The depressive states are the most frequent psychiatric disorders, but so far there has been little attempt to formulate them in learning terms. One difficulty is a nosological one. There is no agreed classification of the depressive disorders. In some, anxiety, depressive and manic illnesses are subsumed under the category of affective disorders (e.g. Lewis, 1966). In addition there is considerable controversy concerning the distinction between endogenous and reactive depression (see Kendall, 1968, for a recent review). Certainly in some depressive states genetic and constitutional factors appear more important than exogenous factors, whereas others appear understandable in terms of a reaction of a particular personality with a particular developmental history to a particular environmental stress. Depressive states are characterized by a combination of subjective emotional experience of misery, self-deprecatory ideas, physiological changes, and overt behavioural manifestations usually in the form of apathy, retardation, or agitation. It has been suggested that this may represent a primary biological reaction to anticipated or actual deprivation which is adaptive in the sense of husbanding resources or feigning death, in contrast with the fear reaction to anticipated or actual danger which prepares the organism for fight or flight. Psychoanalysts have emphasized the adaptive function of mourning in allowing readjustment to occur. Detailed analyses of the genesis and experiential aspects of emotion have been made by many writers (e.g. Shand, 1914; Engel, 1962) and subtle distinctions can be drawn between feelings of guilt, shame, helplessness and hopelessness. Psychoanalytic theory (Abraham, 1911; Freud, 1917) draws a parallel between fear and grief in distinction to anxiety and depression on the basis that the former are responses to external danger and loss whereas the latter are responses to unknown or unconscious danger or loss. Learning theory, on the other hand, is more concerned with the distinction between unconditioned and conditioned emotional responses than the source of the stimuli which evoke them. But it is difficult to concentrate exclusively on the overt behavioural manifestations of depression in considering its aetiology, when pervasive and seemingly excessive guilt feelings are frequently such a prominent feature. Although there are a variety of psychoanalytical formulations of depression, they tend to emphasize the importance of ambivalent feelings the patient has had towards the dead person ('lost object') and the consequent feelings of guilt and self-reproach which can occur, even to the extent of thinking he was responsible for their death and deserves punishment. Certainly bereaved patients often express such ideas, which can reach delusional intensity. In less severe reactions there may be no conscious awareness of hostility and guilt but psychoanalysts consider that these feelings are present at an unconscious level.

There has been much less animal experimentation devoted to the study of depression than to anxiety. One reason for this lies in the uncertainty that there are any animal analogues of human depression. Senay (1966) has discussed possible experimental models and describes an experiment in which some behavioural features of depression appeared in dogs when they no longer had daily contact with him. Hebb (1947) describes a possibly spontaneously occurring 'depressive' state in a chimpanzee. Ethologists have speculated that animals who drop lower in the hierarchy manifest behaviour which bears some resemblance to depression. Whether animal 'hypnotic' states or the 'inhibition' induced in some Pavlovian conditioning experiments has any relationship to depression is highly speculative.

Behaviourists focus on the observed restriction and decrease in behavioural responses. Skinner (1953) considers that weakening of a behavioural repertoire can occur as a result of complete extinction of operant responses (abulia) or an inadequate reinforcement schedule. Ferster (1965) considers that 'depression' may result from a sudden change in the stimulus situation such as the loss of a relative who is the source of generalized reinforcement, or sudden shifts in the contingencies of reinforcement, or punishment by omission of positive reinforcement. Anxiety and depression often coexist and possibly result from the combination of the lack of an effective avoidance response and any positive reinforcement. However, formulations of depression in terms of operant conditioning leave unexplained the drastic reduction in such a wide range of operant responses in the absence of complete elimination of reinforcement or extensive suppression by punishment. Recently, Lazarus (1968a) has adopted a similar theoretical formulation and has described treatment methods for clinical application in depressive states.

In clinical practice, when an environmental situation is found in association with the onset of a depressive state, it is commonly a bereavement or a loss of some significant 'object' such as an important relationship, health, job or money. Increased sensitivity to losses with difficulty in forming new relationships or obtaining alternative sources of reinforcement could be the result of early conditioning. The importance of the affectional tie between mother and baby for the subsequent development of the child has been emphasized by many writers (e.g. Bowlby, 1961). Depressive reaction is one such type of psychiatric disturbance which may result, although there is controversy about its incidence (e.g. W.H.O., 1962; Dennehy, 1966; Granville-Grossman, 1968). In learning terms, the depressive response following bereavement may generalize to other stimuli so that depressive reactions are evoked by a variety of environmental situations which do not directly involve a significant loss. 'Anniversary reactions' in which a recurrence of depression occurs on the anniversary of a bereavement are one common example of a conditioned response.

The aetiology of the sexual deviations remains obscure. Multifactorial causation, with hereditary factors, chromosomal abnormalities, cerebral lesions, endocrine disorders, personality type and environmental factors as possible determinants, is considered likely. A wide variety of sexual behaviour occurs in mammals and man, including prepubertal, homosexual and aggressive activity. This diversity and the differing cultural attitudes towards sexual behaviour suggest that social learning must play a large part in determining the individual's preferred sexual activity. Some learning theorists considered that one trial learning on the basis of the first sexual experience of the individual could determine subsequent sexual interests, because all sexual activity is self-reinforcing. However, if this were so, homosexual behaviour would be more frequent and predominant in adults than is found to be the case. More recently, McGuire *et al.* (1965) have suggested that learning takes place as a result of reinforcement of the masturbatory fantasy preceding orgasm and that the masturbatory fantasy selected is the first real experience of sexual arousal. The advantage of this theory lies in its explanation of the gradual establishment of specific sexually arousing stimuli and the extinction of others. It does not account for the determination of the first sexually arousing stimulus. However, conditioning, both aversive and appetitive, could account for much of the variety in sexual behaviour. Rachman (1966c) has produced an analogue of fetishism by a classical conditioning procedure in which a photograph of black knee-length boots was paired with a photograph of an attractive female nude. Transvestism and exhibitionism may result from similar conditioning experiences. But the strength of the drive for ordinary heterosexual intercourse is sufficiently strong for this to be the predominant sexual activity in the great majority of adults. Where this is not the case the subject may have been exposed to aversive conditioning of heterosexual intercourse as well as positive reinforcement of other sexual responses. Approach behaviour may be in abeyance because of lack of learning (e.g. Harlow's monkeys), or suppression resulting from previous punishment or rejection. Some deviant sexual behaviour appears to have a compulsive quality although it is only rarely accompanied by the subjective characteristics of compulsive experiences. This behavioural similarity has led Metzner (1963) to suggest that some deviant sexual behaviour may become established and fixated if it is both an approach and an avoidance response. 'Compulsive' masturbation could result if other sexual responses had been punished, so that masturbation leads to the avoidance of punished behaviour and reduction of sexual drive simultaneously. In clinical assessment it is helpful to look both for factors which may be inhibiting ordinary heterosexual behaviour and factors which determine the selection of the alternative sexual activity. Male homosexuality, for example, can be analysed both in terms of a sexual phobia of women and sexual attraction to men.

Varying degrees of impotence and frigidity are commonly found in psychiatric disorders. They may occur in association with recognized syndromes such as depressive states or schizophrenia. More often, however, they appear to be either the result of an acute and reversible reaction to a stressful situation or else associated with a more wide-spread neurotic or personality disturbance. In the former case it is often possible to trace the condition to anxiety resulting from aversive conditioning. A previous experience of sexual failure, pain, criticism or guilt and anxiety may be sufficient to condition an anxiety response to subsequent attempts to have intercourse. In those whose impotence or frigidity is accompanied by evidence of other neurotic distur-bances, it is likely that more profound aversive conditioning has been established as a result of punishment and conflict experienced in relationship to heterosexual behaviour and interpersonal relation-ships. This could result in the acquisition of alternative consummatory responses such as homosexuality or a total suppression of overt sexual activity.

Childhood behaviour disorders and adult psychopathic disorders can often be accounted for in terms of operant conditioning. Temper tantrums and other aggressive behaviour may develop as a result of inappropriate reinforcement in which 'constructive' behaviour is un-rewarded and only 'naughty' behaviour receives attention from par-ents or teachers. The child then learns that he can get rewards such as treats and loving attention by being naughty whereas being 'good' is associated with lack of attention and primary rewards. Inconsistent application of reinforcement may cause a child to become anxious or withdrawn if he no longer knows whether he will be punished or rewarded for his behaviour. He is left in a state of ambiguity in which discrimination learning cannot take place. Such situations can lead to intense emotional responses and their endocrine accompaniment (Mason *et al.*, 1966). Childhood is likely to be a vulnerable period because the less well developed state of perception and language will hinder the acquisition of refined discrimination learning.

Adolescent and adult delinquency and psychopathic behaviour may also be maintained by inappropriate schedules of reinforcement. The immediate reward of stolen money or a car and the social approval of his peers may be sufficient to outweigh any delayed punishment in the form of imprisonment or a fine. Most studies of delinquents and psychopaths find a greater than expected incidence of family disturbance in childhood, which suggests that childhood training can be an important factor but does not exclude a genetic influence. Eysenck suggests that psychopaths are neurotic extraverts in whom the combination of emotional reactivity and slow conditioning prevents the acquisition of socially desirable habits. He presents some evidence that psychopaths are characterized by neuroticism and extraversion.

The aetiology of schizophrenia is the major problem in psychiatry today because of its high incidence and the often prolonged suffering and disability it causes. There is no shortage of hypotheses, whether couched mainly in a genetic, neurophysiological, biochemical, psychological or sociological framework. It is impossible to make any statement about aetiology which would not be dissented from by some psychiatrists. However, many would agree that genetic factors can be important, that schizophrenia is occasionally associated with demonstrable cerebral lesions, and that a similar or sometimes seemingly identical clinical syndrome occurs in association with temporal lobe epilepsy, amphetamine intoxication, or following a period of acute or prolonged environmental stress. In comparison with the neurotic disorders, there have been few attempts to present a formulation of schizophrenia in terms of learning principles. This is probably because a majority of behaviour theorists have inclined towards the acceptance of a primarily organic cerebral pathology despite the fact that psychoanalysts, existentialists and social psychiatrists have frequently been able to provide a meaningful account of the content or experience of the schizophrenic's world in terms of previous life experience (e.g. Sullivan, 1955; Jung, 1960; Laing, 1960; Lidz *et al.*, 1966).

However, many psychiatrists have also made a distinction between *nuclear schizophrenia* and *schizophreniform psychoses*. In nuclear schizophrenia, the form of the disorder is considered not to be understandable in terms of the patient's personality and life experience, the prognosis is poor, and a primary cerebral pathology is assumed. In contrast, the schizophreniform psychoses include a variety of disorders whose symptomatology bears some resemblance to schizophrenia but can be understood in terms of the reaction of a particular personality to a particular life experience. The prognosis is better and no primary cerebral pathology is assumed. Obviously, learning processes may be of importance in this type of disorder. But it must be emphasized that there is no clear-cut clinical distinction between 'nuclear schizophrenia' and 'schizophrenia-like' disorders, and the idea that there is a 'true' schizophrenia due to cerebral disease remains a hypothesis.

Schizophrenic patients may show disorders in the spheres of attention, perception, cognition, affect and motivation, in the sense that they do not appear to the observer to be responding appropriately to the external environment. Bleuler (1950) considers that four fundamental symptoms are always present, disturbances of thought association and affectivity, a preference for fantasy over reality, and a tendency to divorce from reality. Dreaming, sensory deprivation, and sleep deprivation can lead to states in which fantasy-dominated autistic thinking with looseness of associations, vivid imagery, delusional ideas and hallucinatory phenomena occur. These conditions, which differ from schizophrenia in some respects but include some aspects of schizophrenic experience, have in common a reduction in external sensory input and a lowering of cerebral arousal. It is postulated that low arousal levels lead to a disturbance of selective attention which results in the emergence of fantasy-dominated internal cues to consciousness. On the other hand, very high levels of cerebral arousal (e.g. panic states or LSD intoxication) also lead to a disorder of selective attention in which the subject appears to be overwhelmed by external sensory stimuli which he fails to filter. It therefore seems likely that there is an optimal level of cerebral arousal for attending to the sensory input of a particular environment and higher or lower levels of arousal interfere with the central processes involved in its organization. The model psychoses associated with decreased sensory input may be examples of too low arousal, whereas the hallucinogenic drug psychoses and schizophrenia may be examples of too high arousal (Luby and Gottlieb, 1968).

Bleuler suggested that many of the symptoms of schizophrenia seem to be an attempt at adaptation to an intolerable situation created by the primary disturbance of disordered association and affectivity. He favoured the hypothesis of a primary cerebral process but did not exclude the possibility that it could be psychically determined. An apparent disregard of or idiosyncratic response to environmental stimuli could be the result of disordered cerebral physiology or perceptual disorders resulting from disorders of the special senses. Chapman (1966), for instance, suggests that subtle disturbances of perception and attention can be detected before the onset of overt schizophrenic symptoms. Hallucinations and paranoid ideation may occur in association with blindness or deafness. However, attention, perception, conceptual thinking and motivation are influenced to a great extent by learning. Therefore schizophrenic experience may also be the result of learning in which the patient reacts to the environment in an apparently inconsistent fashion or by 'escape into fantasy' because the people in his environment have always behaved inconsistently and confusingly towards him or his perception of the environment is distorted. Studies of the early family life of schizophrenic patients and their modes of communication often show disturbed relationships and have led to Bateson's double-bind hypothesis (Bateson *et al.*, 1956), the marital skew and schism described by Lidz, and the relationship between disordered family communication and the type of thought disorder found in the schizophrenic (Singer and Wynne, 1965). It is important to determine the extent to which schizophrenic symptoms can be accounted for as learned responses to such an unfavourable early environment with withdrawal into fantasy as an avoidance response. Recently, Kirk (1968) has put forward a model to account for the schizophrenic state which is thought to be the consequence of the complex interaction which takes place between an unrecognized perceptual defect in the child and the resultant role handicap this induces in his parents.

Operant conditioning techniques have been used to investigate the behavioural repertoire of the schizophrenic patient and the means by which it can be modified. Much of the schizophrenic's behaviour does not appear to be under operant control, because patients are often unresponsive to primary or social reinforcement initially. If the psychotic behaviour is the result of learning, it must have led to devastating and persisting effects to the extent that it has been maintained by the reinforcement contingencies of institutionalization. However, increasing experience of the use of operant conditioning in schizophrenic patients is providing information about their behaviour deficits. Ferster (1961) has been able to improve the behavioural repertoire of autistic children by operant techniques and suggests that autism may occur as the result of the failure of development of secondary and generalized reinforcers when these have not been paired with adequate primary reinforcement.

Skinner and some other writers (Skinner, 1953; Lindsley, 1960; Ferster, 1965) have suggested that all psychiatric symptoms can be traced to inadequate reinforcement histories. Symptoms are conceptualized as operant responses resulting from inadequate or inappropriate reinforcement which prevent the patient from emitting other responses which would allow him to obtain the reinforcements potentially available in his environment. This is an extreme environmentalist approach which has some heuristic value if it leads to a more thorough and exhaustive analysis of the extent to which behaviour is influenced by the reinforcement of overt operant responses. But a careful reading of Skinner's work reveals that the importance of other variables such as heredity and maturation is recognized. If the 'black box' has not been opened explicitly, the treatment of thoughts and feelings as covert operant responses and the hypothetical s–r chains in verbal language are very close to descriptions of central processes or 'mind'. More recently, learning theorists have paid more attention to mediational processes (Osgood, 1953; Mowrer, 1960). s–r theory is s–o–r or s–r–s–r at least. Hebb (1958) has pointed out that until recently learning theorists had paid lip service to the importance of central processes but had treated them in the same way as Jane Austen treated sex in her novels – something very important but not to be spoken about openly. Increasing attention is now being paid to thinking and fantasy (e.g. Hefferline, 1962; Staats and Staats, 1963; Homme, 1965). It is obviously more difficult to investigate the influence of these 'private events' as opposed to the overt behavioural responses of patients but their importance is obvious. Operant conditioning techniques can demonstrably modify or induce 'psychotic behaviour' (Ayllon et al., 1965), but so far only in a proportion of patients and it is usually a very laborious procedure. However, it is fallacious logic to assume that because behaviour can be induced or modified by operant conditioning it must be the consequence of operant conditioning. Davison (1967) has emphasized this point recently and quotes Rimland's (1964) statement that such an inference is as valid as the conclusion that a headache which is relieved by aspirin was caused by lack of aspirin.

In this chapter we have adopted a two-factor learning theory and emphasize mediational processes because they seem to provide a theoretical framework in keeping with experimental and clinical data. As Kimble (1961) points out, it is impossible to separate completely classical and instrumental conditioning procedures. It therefore seems unwise to attempt to account for the development of all behaviour disorders in terms of operant conditioning alone. At times it seems easier to account for psychiatric disorders in terms of genetic or neurophysiological processes but an attempt should also be made to describe them in behavioural terms.

In concluding this chapter we wish to outline some of the strengths, weaknesses, and possible practical applications of aetiological formulations of psychiatric disorder in terms of learning theory. There is no single theory of learning to account for the experimental findings of laboratory learning. Similar data can be accounted for by different theories and crucial experimental tests are often not possible. For example, concepts of habit and drive can often be interchanged with expectancy and value. It follows that a variety of theoretical formulations may encompass the learning of 'abnormal' behaviour as well as that of 'normal' behaviour. Fractional anticipatory responses and mediational processes seem to refer to similar inferred processes. In the present state of learning theory it is misleading to suggest that the behaviour therapists' formulation of psychiatric disorder is derived from an established 'modern learning theory'. To the extent that it is derived from any single theoretical orientation, it runs the risk of having a restricted application.

The hypothesis that neurotic or other psychiatric symptoms are learned patterns of behaviour remains a hypothesis. It receives some support from animal laboratory experiments in which behaviour reminiscent of human neurosis can be induced and modified by conditioning procedures in a proportion of animals. Some acute traumatic neuroses in humans bear a resemblance to animal experimental neuroses. Learning processes can modify existing psychiatric symptoms. However, none of these findings provides direct evidence that psychiatric disorders are due primarily to learning. It is certain that genetic and organic processes are necessary and sufficient causes of some psychiatric disorders and it is impossible to exclude them from being involved in some of the 'functional' psychiatric disorders.

Formulations derived from laboratory animal experiments based solely on a behavioural analysis must almost certainly be too restricted to account for the diversity of human behaviour. The animal model of 'neurotic' behaviour rests heavily on aversive conditioning and the concept of conditioned fear. The effect of the prolonged period of dependency and maturation in childhood and the special opportunity this might afford for adverse experiences to influence personality development and adult behaviour does not receive emphasis. Similarly, it seems very unlikely that the presence of language, conceptual processes and fantasy does not play a significant role in human learning and behaviour. Schachter (1964), for instance, has demonstrated the influence of cognitive factors on the individual's identification of emotional states. Internal responses such as tachycardia may be recognized as joy or anger according to the prevailing environmental factors. The complex social organization of man is also unlikely to be an irrelevant variable in the determination of his behaviour. Some learning theorists have tended to neglect individual differences in personality.

As clinical experience in behaviour therapy has accumulated, behaviour therapists have become more and more aware of the limitations of their original theoretical models. Psychiatric disorder can manifest itself in any type of behaviour and subjective experience. It is therefore important to consider the whole body of experimental psychology including cognition, perception and motivation as well as learning processes. Nor is it sensible to disregard the body of knowledge accumulated in the related disciplines of neurophysiology, biochemistry and pharmacology. None of these criticisms of behaviour therapy theory should lead to its outright rejection. It will certainly need modification but there is much to be said in favour of starting with as simple a model as possible and ascertaining how far it can account for seemingly more complex phenomena. Behaviour theory has already proved a stimulus to fruitful research and the reassessment of existing therapeutic methods.

It is easier to account for discrete symptoms such as isolated phobias in terms of learning principles than to account for the complex neuroses and personality disorders. But it does not follow from this, as some writers imply (e.g. Fish, 1964), that learning processes are not involved in their development. Higher-order conditioning, generalization, response-produced cues and avoidance responses can account for 'repression', 'underlying conflicts' and disturbances in interpersonal relationships found in many neurotic disorders. It is possible to provide a linguistic bridge between various learning theory constructs and psychoanalytical theory as Dollard and Miller have done. This has led some psychotherapists to point out that behaviour therapists are rediscovering 'well-established psychodynamic principles'. In a sense this is true and not surprising. Both are attempting to account for the same clinical phenomena. They both take cognizance of constitutional predisposition and developmental history and try to relate current psychiatric symptoms to the interaction between the patient and his environment. As already mentioned, the main differences are that behaviour therapists do not postulate that the Oedipus complex is a universal psychic conflict or that it is always the major source of conflict in adult life. They do not consider that the form of an adult neurosis is always determined by childhood experience, whereas psychoanalytic theory maintains that only the actual (traumatic) neuroses in adults are not determined by childhood experience.

Apart from these theoretical considerations there are differences of emphasis in approach. The behaviourist is more likely to look for the relationship between current symptoms and the environmental stimuli upon which they are contingent. A behavioural approach may lead more quickly to the identification of the particular stress to which the present symptom is a learned response. However, it is not always possible to trace the development of the symptoms with any degree of confidence. The aetiology of psychiatric disorders appears to be extremely complex and the available knowledge is limited. Sufficient evidence has been adduced, however, that learning principles offer a distinct contribution to our understanding of the development and persistence of behavioural abnormalities.

Chapter 4

Theory and Methods of Treatment

Since behaviour therapy conceptualizes psychiatric disorders as learned patterns of behaviour, learning principles should serve as the necessary guidance for treatment. Direct modification of symptoms is attempted by the process of unlearning maladaptive and learning adaptive responses. At present it is difficult to classify the various methods of treatment in a satisfactory way. This is partly a result of confusion in terminology. The same technique may be named according to its assumed theoretical basis or the operations involved. In this chapter some of the main methods of treatment in behaviour therapy are described. The classification adopted is a descriptive one, but the postulated processes which underlie them are discussed.

Conditioning of incompatible responses

Treatment methods included in this category aim to establish acceptable and adaptive responses to stimuli which previously evoked symptoms. The underlying principle involved is that of *counter-conditioning* in which the acquisition and strengthening of a new response, incompatible with the existing response to the stimulus, leads to the elimination of the old response. Treatment techniques based on counter-conditioning have been used extensively in a wide range of neurotic conditions.

Direct retraining in real-life situations

Mary Cover Jones's studies (1924a and b) of the treatment of children with phobias demonstrated the value of direct 'deconditioning' of anxiety and paved the way for the development of more advanced techniques for dealing with symptoms mediated by anxiety. The treatment of Peter, who had a fear of rabbits, illustrates the procedure.

Peter was given some food and the experimenter brought a rabbit in a cage into the room, but at such a distance that Peter continued eating. The cage was gradually brought closer and the rabbit was released from the cage while Peter was still eating. The fear response to the rabbit was replaced by eating in the presence of the rabbit. Initially the positive feeding response can only be elicited when the feared object is at a distance. Gradually, as a result of stimulus generalization, eating could take place when the rabbit was brought close.

The principle of establishing a response antagonistic to anxiety by means of graduated stages in which the intensity or proximity of the original fearful stimulus is increased has been used for the treatment of irrational fears in children (Jersild and Holmes, 1935) and phobias in adult patients (Meyer, 1957; Meyer and Gelder, 1963; Marks and Gelder, 1965; Gelder and Marks, 1966). The method, sometimes called gradual habituation or toleration, involves the graduated exposure to the actual feared situation or object. Often no special effort is made to establish a specific response antagonistic to anxiety. It is assumed that the presence of the therapist is sufficient to produce feelings of comfort in the patient which will be incompatible with anxiety. Agoraphobics are required to walk gradually increasing distances at first accompanied by the therapist and then by themselves. Claustrophobics are placed in rooms of gradually smaller size. A patient with a phobia of cats was presented with the following hierarchy of stimuli: materials graded in texture and appearance from very unlike to very like cat fur; a toy kitten; pictures of cats; a live kitten which the patient eventually took home to keep (Freeman and Kendrick, 1960). It was expected that the non-anxiety response to the kitten would strengthen and generalize to other kittens and cats.

When treatment by practical retraining is undertaken, a careful history is taken from the patient so that all the important anxiety-provoking stimuli can be identified and graded according to intensity. A hierarchy of stimuli is then compiled with the patient ranking the items according to the amount of anxiety experienced with each.

Systematic desensitization in imagination

Wolpe (1958) developed a variety of treatment methods based on the principle that 'If a response antagonistic to anxiety can be made to occur in the presence of anxiety-evoking stimuli so that it is accompanied by a complete or partial suppression of the anxiety response, the bond between these stimuli and the anxiety responses will be weakened.' The procedure involves the counter-conditioning of responses which are incompatible with anxiety. In order to account for this principle, Wolpe put forward the more general concept of 'reciprocal inhibition', a term first used by Sherrington in relation to spinal reflexes. Wolpe extended this to include higher neurophysiological processes – any situation 'in which the elicitation of one response appears to bring about a decrement in the strength of evocation of a simultaneous response'. He further suggested that if the incompatible response was followed by drive reduction, conditioned inhibition of the original response would occur.

Wolpe has suggested several responses which are incompatible with anxiety and has developed a number of treatment techniques associated with the principle of reciprocal inhibition. Of the various behavioural responses considered antagonistic to anxiety, muscular relaxation has been the most extensively employed and forms the basis of the 'systematic desensitization' of symptoms mediated by anxiety. This method has an advantage over retraining *in vivo* in that it can be carried out in the consulting room, and therefore avoids the more time-consuming and often difficult procedure of finding suitably graded anxiety stimuli in real-life situations.

Only a brief description of the operations involved in systematic desensitization will be given, since detailed accounts have already been published (Wolpe, 1961; Wolpe and Lazarus, 1966). We may take as an example an isolated phobia of spiders. A detailed history is obtained from the patient with particular attention directed towards those characteristics of the phobic stimulus which influence the intensity of the anxiety it evokes. With a spider, the relevant dimensions may be size, colour, movement and proximity, so that the larger, darker, more active and nearer the spider is, the more intense the anxiety aroused. From this information it should be possible to construct a graded hierarchy of items from those evoking minimal anxiety such as a small, light, still spider five yards from the patient, to items which arouse intense anxiety, such as a large, black, active spider touching the patient's face. The items are written on separate slips of paper and the patient is asked to rank them in order. The construction of the hierarchy is usually completed in one to three interviews.

During the initial interviews the patient is trained in muscular relaxation, usually an abbreviated form of Jacobson's method (1938), in which the patient first contracts and then relaxes particular muscle groups while he learns to appreciate the difference in sensation between tense and relaxed muscles. The patient is usually asked to practise relaxation at home between treatment sessions. There is some variation among therapists in the actual technique employed to attain relaxation. Some therapists make use of hypnotic suggestion (Wolpe, 1958; Stafford Clark, 1963) or some modification of autogenic training (Schultz and Luthe, 1959). However, hypnosis is not an essential requirement, and may be omitted in patients who are not easily hypnotized or who object to it.

When a 'sufficient' degree of relaxation has been obtained, desensitization is started. The patient is asked to relax in the way he has learned and is told to signal by raising his index finger whenever he feels anxious or disturbed. He is then asked to imagine a neutral scene which does not evoke anxiety, and this is followed by the presentation of one or two of the lowest items of the anxiety hierarchy. During the first session of desensitization an attempt is made to discover how quickly and vividly the patient is able to imagine the items and how he feels when imagining them. At subsequent sessions a similar basic procedure is adhered to. It is customary to start with the most difficult item in the hierarchy which had no longer aroused anxiety in the previous session. If this does not arouse anxiety, the next item is presented and the procedure is repeated until the strongest anxiety-provoking stimulus can be imagined without any anxiety.

Lazarus (1964) has drawn attention to 'crucial procedural factors' and provided 'a logical and consistent *modus operandi*' for desensitization. The most important point is to maintain deep relaxation throughout the sessions to prevent the desensitization process itself acquiring anxiety-mediating properties. If the patient signals anxiety or the therapist observes any signs of bodily disturbance during presentation of the first item, the patient is told to stop imagining the item and to relax deeply again. Sometimes, in addition, the patient is asked to imagine a peaceful scene which is conducive to feelings of calm. The item is then presented again. If anxiety is still aroused, deep relaxation is reinstated, and the hierarchy is extended to include weaker items which can be successfully presented to the patient. The occurrence of repeated anxiety to a particular stimulus is handled by presenting again items which have already been mastered. If the new item continues to evoke anxiety, it is necessary to construct extra items in the hierarchy which are midway in 'strength' between the previous one and the difficult one, so that desensitization can proceed in more gradual stages. No session should end with a period of anxiety, because the last item of any learning series is retained well, and it may require a longer time for the anxiety to extinguish. Because of this, it is customary to present an easier item at the end of the session.

During the early presentation of items the scene is imagined for several seconds. This is increased in subsequent exposures until it has been held for about fifteen seconds without anxiety. Obviously there is some variation in the time according to how long it takes the patient to conjure up a vivid image of the scene. The duration it should be held will depend to some extent on the nature of the scene. A brief exposure might be sufficient for a flash of lightning whereas a scene involving a half-mile walk would need to be imagined for several minutes. The interval between the presentation of items is usually a few seconds if no anxiety was evoked, or the time taken to reinstate relaxation if anxiety had been evoked.

There are no fixed rules for the number of items presented in a single session or for its duration. The availability of time and the endurance of the patient are the main determining factors. Initial sessions usually last twenty to thirty minutes two or three times a week. Wolpe (1961) states that whether sessions are massed together or widely spaced, there is almost always a close relationship between the extent to which desensitization has been accomplished and the degree of diminution of anxiety responses to real stimuli. One study (Ramsay et al., 1966), however, indicates that distributed practice conditions may be more efficient.

In most patients the stimuli which arouse excess anxiety fall into separate groups according to their underlying theme and it is necessary to construct more than one anxiety hierarchy. If this is the case, it is usual to present a few items from each hierarchy during a single session.

Desensitization in imagination has usually been carried out individually with each patient. More recently, Lazarus (1961b, 1968e) has described the group desensitization of patients. Patients with the same type of phobia (e.g. claustrophobia) were all given the same hierarchy for desensitization. A group with different phobias were handed the items of their own hierarchy on slips of paper. Paul and Shannon (1966) and Kondas (1967a) employed group desensitization for subjects with fears of public speaking and examinations.

Recently Migler and Wolpe (1967) introduced 'automated desensitization' in the treatment of a patient with a fear of public speaking. Relaxation and desensitization instructions were recorded in the patient's own voice on a specially modified tape recorder. The patient took the tape recorder home and administered the desensitization sessions himself. Wolpe reports that Lang treated several subjects with a fear of snakes by tape recorder.

Desensitization has usually been carried out in imagination alone. Sometimes, however, it has been combined with graded retraining *in vivo*, or desensitization under relaxation with the presentation of real stimuli has been performed (Marks and Gelder, 1965; Meyer and Crisp, 1966).

Some therapists have used drugs instead of or as an adjunct to Jacobson's method of muscle relaxation. Wolpe has suggested the use of tranquillizers such as meprobamate and chlorpromazine, and has used codeine phosphate. Premedication with pethidine and scopolamine has been used by Rachman (1957). Lazarus (1959) has employed amylobarbitone and phenalglycodal in children, and Friedman (1966a) uses a rapid acting barbiturate, methohexitone sodium, in subanaesthetic doses. The advantages claimed for the latter procedure include its rapidity of action, absence of sedative after-effects, and the ease of control of the depth of relaxation by retaining the intravenous needle in the vein throughout desensitization so that the drug can be administered as necessary.

Muscular relaxation, with or without drugs as adjuncts, has been the most frequently employed response in systematic desensitization. Less commonly used techniques include the use of emotive imagery, feeding, sexual, assertive and 'anxiety relief' responses. Lazarus (1959) utilized feeding responses in the treatment of children's phobias.

Lazarus and Abramovitz (1962) reported the use of 'emotive imagery' capable of arousing positive feelings.

Two other kinds of responses considered by Wolpe to be incompatible with anxiety have been exploited therapeutically. Sexual responses have been used to antagonize the anxiety which is thought to underlie sexual disorders such as partial impotence. The patient is prohibited from attempting sexual intercourse unless he experiences strong sexual arousal and penile erection. If the patient is able to follow out these instructions, the anticipatory anxiety previously experienced in 'sexual situations' should no longer occur, because, when intercourse is attempted under strong sexual arousal, anxiety is inhibited. When impotence is complete and anxiety is sufficiently strong to prevent sexual arousal in the real-life situation, systematic desensitization in imagination can be carried out prior to the use of sexual responses in practical retraining.

'Assertive' responses are also thought by Wolpe to be antagonistic to anxiety. Where anxiety is experienced in interpersonal situations, as, for example, when being criticized unfairly, the patient is trained to respond assertively but appropriately. Assertive responses are carried out in progressively more demanding or stressful real-life situations. Assertive training can be combined with systematic desensitization. When the subject is quite unable to initiate appropriate assertive responses in real life, he can practise them first in the consulting room with the therapist playing the part of a person who usually evokes anxiety. After rehearsal of this 'psychodrama' until anxiety is no longer experienced, inhibition of anxiety is expected to generalize to the real-life situation. Relaxation may be induced if anxiety is aroused even in the performance of the psychodrama. Lazarus (1966a) has used a role-playing technique which he terms 'behavioural rehearsal'.

Although the use of sexual and assertive responses have been included under the heading of desensitization in imagination, it will be seen that they are employed also in role playing and real life situations.

Anxiety relief technique

In the search for other suitable responses which might be antagonistic to anxiety, Wolpe has used experimentally induced 'anxiety relief' responses. The principle underlying this technique is that if the termination of a noxious stimulus follows immediately after some other stimulus, the presentation of this stimulus alone will be followed by relief of anxiety. Wolpe's original application of the method involved the administration of an electric shock to the patient's forearm. The patient could terminate the shock when it became too painful by saying the word 'calm'. After many such trials, the patient found that saying the word 'calm' in other situations induced a feeling of relief. He was then instructed to use the word whenever he felt disturbed in everyday situations.

Until recently only isolated cases using this technique have been reported (Meyer, 1957; Lazarus, 1959, 1963). However, Solyom and Miller (1967) have published the results of a modified technique in a small sample of phobic patients. Phobic stimuli were presented to the patient simultaneously with the elicitation of a 'relief' response – pressing a button to terminate an electroshock. Each patient had written an account of the anxiety-producing situations which was then tape-recorded and played to the patient during the treatment session. A silence of thirty seconds was followed by the administration of the shock. When the patient pressed the button to terminate the shock, the taped phobic stimulus was presented. The sequence for a patient with a cat phobia might be 'As I walk down the street' . . . thirty second pause, electric shock . . . button pressed, 'I see a cat' . . . thirty second pause, electric shock . . . button pressed, 'and feel my heart begin to pound. . . .' Several tapes describing variations in the phobic situation were used. Initially every pause was followed by a shock, but then partial reinforcement with a 70–80 per cent schedule was introduced. With the latter schedule, termination of the pause itself elicited relief. Obviously, visual as well as auditory stimuli can be used and this method of treatment can be combined with practical retraining in real life.

In a preliminary communication Kushner (1967) has reported on the use of an automated 'anxiety relief' procedure. A tape was programmed to give an uncomfortable electric shock to the fingertip on a variable interval schedule. The shock was terminated by the patient saying 'calm' into a microphone which activated the voice key. Patients can be 'treated' by this procedure without the therapist being present. This method has been introduced as an alternative for patients with anxiety states which failed to respond to systematic desensitization methods.

Imitation

Autonomic and instrumental responses can be acquired as a result of social imitation. However, until recently there have been few attempts to employ imitation learning in a systematic fashion in the treatment of patients. There is some evidence that conditioned emotional responses can be extinguished by having the subject observe a model behaving in a relaxed manner in the presence of the feared object. Early attempts at vicarious extinction of phobias produced variable results (Bandura, 1965b). Bandura argues that this may have been due to the generation of very high levels of anxiety in the observer when the model was seen in the most fearful situation at the outset of treatment, and a high anxiety level would impede vicarious extinction.

Bandura and his colleagues (Bandura *et al.*, 1967; Bandura and Menlove, 1968; Bandura, 1968) have explored further the therapeutic value of vicarious extinction of avoidance behaviour in children and adults with fears of dogs or snakes. In a series of experiments they have refined the technique so that the subjects observe the model in a graded series of anxiety-producing situations with the model gradually displaying longer, closer and more active interaction with the dog. Muscular relaxation may be induced in the subject and maintained throughout the observation of the model's behaviour and the rate of presentation may be controlled by the subject himself. The observation of live models is more effective than films. When the subject is unable to overcome his fear by observation alone, he is encouraged to participate gradually in the fearless behaviour of the model.

Positive conditioning

Enuresis. The methods of counter-conditioning described so far have been concerned with elimination of anxiety in patients whose symptoms are thought to be mediated by anxiety. However, counter-conditioning techniques may also be employed to establish instrumental responses. The best-known example of this is the treatment of nocturnal enuresis, in which inhibition of micturition during sleep has to be established. One commonly used method is the bell and pad (Mowrer and Mowrer, 1938). The pad is placed under the sheet on which the patient lies. When he wets the bed, the bell rings, wakes him, and micturition is inhibited until he reaches the lavatory. In terms of classical conditioning the bell is the UCS, bladder distension the CS, and waking and sphincter contraction the response. After several trials the stimulus of bladder distension alone is sufficient to evoke sphincter contraction.

Crosby (1950) has used an apparatus which delivers an electric shock to the loin as soon as the bed is wet. He has suggested that the wet urinous state ('somatic discomfort') acts as the stimulus which inhibits micturition and that conditioning treatments produce their effect by increasing the somatic discomfort. Jones (1960) offered a detailed analysis of treatment in terms of the development of cortical 'sentinel points'. He argued that there were no essential differences between Mowrer's and Crosby's techniques. Crosby's method has the disadvantage of being potentially more traumatic to the child.

Lovibond (1964) has reviewed the theoretical basis and conditioning methods employed in enuresis. He is critical of the classical conditioning model proposed to account for the efficacy of the bell and pad method on the grounds that the conditioned stimulus (bladder distension) is not neutral in relation to the conditioned response of sphincter contraction. In addition, classically conditioned reflexes usually extinguish quickly whereas the bell and pad method can produce a lasting cure of enuresis. Lovibond has suggested that the treatment is an example of traumatic avoidance learning in which noise or electrical stimulation are noxious stimuli (UCS) which elicit the avoidance response of sphincter contraction, and sphincter relaxation, not bladder distension, is the conditioned stimulus. During treatment sphincter relaxation is followed by an aversive stimulus of noise or shock and so becomes the conditioned stimulus of the avoidance response. In order to facilitate such conditioning, the response of sphincter contraction should terminate both the noxious stimulus and the conditioned stimulus. Lovibond constructed a 'twin signal' instrument which emits a loud tone when urination occurs. The signal lasts for just less than a second, which is slightly longer than the latency of the response of sphincter contraction, so that the response leads to escape from both the noxious and the conditioned stimulus. The first signal is followed by a silent interval of about one minute and then a buzzer sounds until it is switched off. The purpose of the buzzer is to summon an attendant to dry the pad and change the sheet.

Lovibond has experimented with various schedules of intermittent reinforcement in an attempt to increase the resistance to extinction of bladder control, and Young and Turner (1965) have reported on the use of methedrine which increases the speed of conditioning in some patients but can also lead to a higher extinction rate. These are discussed in chapter 5.

Stammering. Positive conditioning methods have been used in an attempt to establish normal speech in stammerers. The aetiology of this disorder is uncertain, but both constitutional and psychological factors probably play some part. Anxiety conditioned to the act of speaking could be a causal factor and the stammer which is much worse or only occurs in stressful social situations provides some evidence for this. However, although anxiety can both disrupt speech and motivate avoidance responses such as hesitations and repetitions, it does not offer a completely adequate explanation of the condition (Yates, 1963). Behaviour therapy aimed at reduction of anxiety by desensitization and other techniques have not met with much success in eliminating stammer.

It has been found that manipulation of the subject's own perception of speech can both induce and relieve 'stammering'. Delayed auditory feedback (DAF) in which the subject's speech is relayed back to him through headphones with a delay of 0·18 seconds disrupts normal speech. Elimination of stammering has sometimes been accomplished by methods which alter auditory feedback. Cherry and Sayers (1956) introduced the technique of 'shadowing', in which the patient repeats aloud the speech of the experimenter or a tape recording, one or two words behind. Inhibition of stammering can also occur in simultaneous reading aloud or when auditory feedback is suppressed by a loud masking tone. The clinical application of shadowing techniques have been reported by Marland (1956), MacLaren (1960) and Kondas (1967b), but have seldom been used as the sole basis of treatment.

Other methods of treating stammering make use of the empirical finding that most patients can very quickly master syllabic or rhythmic speech. Andrews *et al.* (1964) trained child stutterers in syllabic speech and instructed them to use this pattern of speech in everyday situations. The original observation which served as the rationale for Meyer and Mair's (1963) technique was the claim that an externally imposed rhythm (usually supplied by a metronome) would eliminate stammer in most patients when they were instructed to speak in time with the beat. However, this technique led to improvement only during the treatment session. Outside the consulting room, where the stresses might be greater and control could not be exerted, most patients were unable to speak rhythmically. In order to overcome this difficulty, a portable electronic apparatus which could be worn behind the ear was used. The instrument produces audible clicks whose frequency and amplitude can be adjusted. With this a graduated training programme falling into four stages was adopted. The first stage involves training the patient with the metronome and determining the optimal beat frequency. In the second stage the patient wears the apparatus and is instructed to speak with it in progressively more stressful situations in everyday life. In the third stage, when sufficient confidence has been gained, he is required to switch off the instrument but to continue speaking as if it were still functioning. Gradually he may revert to a normal rate and manner of speech. If anxiety or difficulty is encountered or anticipated, the instrument must be switched on again. In the final stage, when periods of fluency with the instrument switched off have been achieved, it is removed altogether. If any difficulty is encountered at this stage, speech must be slowed down to a rhythmic pattern again. If this is not sufficient, the apparatus is worn again and switched on if necessary. Obviously the incorporation of a graduated training programme in this method might allow reciprocal inhibition of anxiety to develop, but the reason why rhythm can exert active control over stammering remains uncertain. It does not appear to act merely as a distractor because arhythmic beats do not improve stuttering (Fransella and Beech, 1965; Fransella, 1967). Furthermore the efficacy of the metronome cannot be accounted for entirely by the simple slowing down of the stammerer's speech.

Frequency of micturition. Another example of positive conditioning achieved by alteration of perceptual feedback is furnished by an ingenious technique used by Jones (1956) to treat a patient with frequency of micturition resulting from anxiety. The urge to micturate usually occurs at a particular internal bladder pressure for each individual. When a manometer recording the pressure is connected so that it is visible to the subject, a conditioned reflex of micturition can be established to the pressure reading so that the urge to urinate could be evoked by calling out the critical bladder pressure. Jones used a similar apparatus with his patient, but falsified the manometer readings so that increasingly large amounts of urine collected in the bladder without raising the pressure reading seen by the patient.

Involuntary movements. The rationale underlying the treatment of various involuntary movements such as tics, cramps and torticollis is similar to the other methods of positive conditioning already described. Relaxation exercises aimed at the immobilization of the muscles involved in the abnormal movements are combined with training in the performance of active muscular responses which are incompatible with the execution of the abnormal responses.

Aversion therapy

Aversion therapy is perhaps both the best known and the most controversial form of behaviour therapy. It has been employed mainly in the treatment of approach responses which can be disadvantageous to the individual and which usually also incur social disapproval. Alcoholism, drug addiction, homosexuality, transvestism and fetishism are the conditions most often treated with aversion techniques. The principle underlying treatment is the creation of a conditioned aversion to the undesired habit either by applying a noxious stimulus when the act is performed or by pairing a noxious stimulus with the cues which usually evoke the behaviour. The rationale of aversion treatment is that a conditioned anxiety response will become associated with the undesired behaviour and its cues and will lead to the establishment of an incompatible response. It seems legitimate to consider aversion therapy as another example of conditioning of incompatible responses.

A large number of aversion techniques have been used. In this section we can only outline some of them. Detailed reviews of the treatment of alcoholism and sexual disorders have been published by Franks (1966) and Feldman (1966). Until recently the emetic drugs, emetine and apomorphine, were the most frequently employed aversive stimuli. In one method the alcoholic is taken into a room in which there is a bar with bottles of liquor prominently displayed. He is given an injection of emetine hydrochloride (the emetic), pilocarpine (to induce sweating and salivation) and ephedrine (to prevent any dangerous fall in blood pressure). He is also given an oral dose of emetine in saline which is supposed to cause gastric irritation and to increase the quantity of fluid in the stomach to be regurgitated. When the patient starts to feel sick he is urged to smell and taste a selection of his favourite drinks, particularly when the nausea reaches its height. A large vomiting bowl is provided. Aversive treatment sessions are usually given daily at first, followed by 'booster' treatments at irregular intervals to try to prevent relapse. Between the treatment sessions the patient is encouraged to take soft drinks freely, so that discrimination between alcoholic and non-alcoholic beverages is established. Some therapists have used this procedure in the treatment of groups of alcoholic patients.

Similar aversion methods have been employed in the treatment of sexual deviations. During the period of induced nausea, homosexuals may be shown photographs of male nudes which they have previously selected as being sexually attractive. Transvestites and fetishists may be shown photographs of their sexually preferred objects, or actually cross-dress or handle the fetish object. Sometimes additional 'aids' have been used. The fantasies which accompany the real experiences may be reinforced verbally by the therapist during treatment. Tape-recordings describing the patient's behaviour and its harmful effects may be used during the treatment session and played between sessions as well.

Aversion treatment of sexual deviations may be combined with attempts to stimulate heterosexual interest by showing photographs or films of attractive females. Obviously, aversion treatment by itself aims at inhibiting a particular pattern of response. Its replacement by more adaptive responses cannot always be expected to follow automatically. Other methods of treatment may have to be used for this.

Many therapists follow up the aversion treatment of alcoholism with maintenance treatment with disulfiram (antabuse), a drug which interferes with the normal metabolism of alcohol. A patient who drinks any alcohol while taking disulfiram will develop a severe reaction with flushing, headache, nausea and vomiting. This is a direct physiological reaction due to interaction of the drug with alcohol. However, the patient who has taken his disulfiram tablet in the morning knows that he will have the reaction if he does drink. In that sense a new association between alcohol and the unpleasant reaction may be established which can help to prevent drinking.

There are many disadvantages attached to the use of emetic drugs in aversion treatment and they are now used less frequently. Emetine and apomorphine have toxic side effects and fatalities have occurred with their use. Patients who are in poor physical health have to be excluded from treatment. Apomorphine has an hypnotic action which might impair the conditioning process, but a more important factor which impedes conditioning is the uncertainty of the time of onset, intensity and duration of nausea. In classical conditioning, the inter-stimulus interval should be precisely controlled, and this is virtually impossible to achieve when emetine or apomorphine are used. In the methods described above, the CS has followed the UCS, and backward conditioning is less effective. Eysenck (1968a) has suggested that it is the link between the CS and the UCR rather than that between the CS and UCS which may be of critical importance in aversive conditioning. He gives as an example the treatment of alcoholism with emetic drugs in which the injection of the drug is given before the CS (alcohol). According to Eysenck, this would be a case of backward conditioning with the UCS presented before the CS. However, it is questionable whether the injection *per se* should be considered as the UCS for nausea. It seems more reasonable to regard the afferent stimulation of the vomiting centre as the UCS, in which case the UCS and UCR are experienced nearly simultaneously. But is still important to know the time of onset of the UCS–UCR for successful conditioning to be established.

These considerations have led to attempts to circumvent the difficulties involved with these techniques. Raymond (1964) employed apomorphine in the treatment of alcoholics, but spent the first few sessions in determining the minimal dose required to produce nausea and its exact time of onset. The patient is given a small amount of alcohol to drink immediately before nausea is expected and is stopped from drinking as soon as the nausea starts to subside.

Sanderson *et al.* (1963, 1964) carried out experimental studies to assess the efficacy of drug-induced muscle and respiratory paralysis as an aversive stimulus in the treatment of alcoholism. The drug employed was succinyl choline (scoline), which, when given intravenously, produces total muscle paralysis, without any impairment of consciousness, for a period of sixty to ninety seconds. The patient remains completely aware of his environment but is unable to breathe, speak or move. The scoline was injected into an intravenous saline infusion which had already been set up, immediately after the patient had looked at and sniffed his usual alcoholic drink. He was given a small sip just before the expected onset of paralysis. Further experience with this technique has now been published and will be referred to in the next two chapters.

The modifications of the traditional pharmacological methods of aversion are an improvement, but they still have many drawbacks. Because of this, several workers have advocated the use of electric shock as the aversive stimulus (e.g. Barker, 1965; Rachman, 1965a). Its advantages include the much more precise control of the timing, intensity and duration of the stimulus, and the possibility of using partial reinforcement. In addition, the risk of dangerous side effects is much less, fewer patients have to be excluded because of physical illness, and the treatment is much less unpleasant for the patient, therapist and nursing staff. A note of caution has been sounded by Wilson and Davison (1969) concerning the indiscriminate selection of aversive stimuli for conditioning. They quote some experimental and clinical evidence showing that taste stimuli are more readily conditioned to an UCS of nausea than of electric shock, while auditory, visual and tactile CS are more readily conditioned to the electric shock. If this is confirmed, attention will have to be given to the appropriateness of the aversive stimulus. If an aversion to the smell and taste of alcohol is required, an olfactory, gustatory or nauseating UCS may be more effective than electric shock.

98

Conditioning of incompatible responses

A large variety of procedures using electric shock in a classical conditioning paradigm have been reported. The recommended shock device should apply a relatively high voltage (85–150 volts), and deliver a very low constant current of 0·005 amps or less (Fried, 1967). It is usual to determine the discomfort and the pain thresholds for electrical stimulation before each treatment session, and to employ intensities between these thresholds as the noxious stimulus. In the treatment of homosexuals, electric shock has been paired with photographs of male nudes (e.g. Thorpe and Schmidt, 1964; Thorpe et al., 1964a), and with sexually stimulating words presented tachistoscopically (Thorpe et al., 1964b). Similar techniques have been employed in other forms of sexual deviation. With alcoholics, the sight, smell and taste of alcohol as well as words and suggestions normally associated with drinking have been paired with electric shock. In other procedures the patient is required to imagine vividly his deviant act or the fantasies which accompany it, and to signal to the therapist when the image is clear so that the shock can be delivered (e.g. Max, 1935; McGuire and Vallance 1964). Although often described in terms of classical conditioning, this last procedure could be considered an example of operant conditioning in so far as the UCS is contingent on the patient's fantasy response. McGuire and Vallance (1964) have designed a small portable electric apparatus which the patient can take home. He administers shocks to himself whenever he is tempted to indulge in the sexual fantasy concerned. Another form of self-treatment has been reported in a preliminary communication by Kushner (1967). Alcoholics can administer a shock to the fingertips when presented with tape-recorded stimuli associated with their drinking.

The majority of therapists have used classical conditioning models in the attempt to associate fear with the inappropriate attractive stimuli. However, the disorders of behaviour treated by aversion include overt instrumental responses as well as mediational components, and these responses can be submitted to behavioural modification. In fact instrumental conditioning may be a more appropriate method of treatment because experimental evidence suggests that avoidance conditioning is more resistant to extinction than classical conditioning. Feldman (1966), in a detailed discussion of aversion techniques, has advocated the use of instrumental escape or avoidance learning in which escape from or avoidance of the aversive stimulus is contingent upon withdrawal from the previously attractive stimuli.

Several techniques employing the escape learning paradigm have been used. Blakemore *et al.* (1963) treated a transvestite by requiring him to cross-dress in his favourite female clothes and observe himself in a mirror (the act from which he derived maximum pleasure) while he was standing on an electrified grid which could administer an unpleasant electric shock to the feet. At some time during the cross-dressing procedure either a series of electric shocks or buzzing sounds would be administered until the patient had undressed completely. In half the trials shock was given and in half the buzzer was used. The treatment was randomized so that the patient would not know which signal he would receive or at which point in the cross-dressing it would start. Five trials, with a one-minute interval between them, were given at half-hourly intervals over a six-day period. A total of four hundred trials were given.

Marks and Gelder (1967) have treated transvestites and fetishists by giving a warning signal from one to one-hundred-and-twenty seconds after the patient had started to cross-dress or handle the fetish object. One to three electric shocks were given at random intervals after this, stopping when all the articles had been discarded. An intermittent reinforcement schedule was used, with shocks not given in 25 per cent of the trials. The authors also introduced 'fantasy trials' in which the patient was required to signal as soon as he had a clear image of a given aspect of the deviant behaviour. The signal was followed by one or two shocks which dispelled the image.

Similar methods of escape training have been employed in the treatment of obesity and alcoholism. Meyer and Crisp (1964) administered electric shocks to two obese patients at some stage during their approach to or eating of favourite foods. The shocks were stopped as soon as the patient pushed the food away or stopped eating it. As avoidance behaviour became established, the patient was exposed to the tempting food for progressively longer periods while the frequency of shocks was diminished. Blake (1965) has treated alcoholics by administering a shock of increasing intensity after they had started to sip alcohol and before they had swallowed it. The shock was terminated when the alcohol was spat out. Blake employed a 50 per cent random reinforcement schedule, a green light being used as the signal to spit out in the non-reinforced trials. Hsu (1965) used a combined 'operant and classical conditioning situation' in which alcoholics were presented with a tray containing glasses of beer, wine, whisky, milk, water and fruit juice which they were instructed to drink in whichever order they preferred. A shock was automatically given whenever one of the alcoholic drinks was taken. In the fourth session the patient was asked to drink any five of the six beverages, and in the next session any four out of the six.

Further modifications of aversion therapy have resulted from careful consideration of the theoretical basis of the nature and effect of punishment. There are both semantic and psychophysiological aspects involved. As already mentioned in chapter 2, Mowrer (1950) has pointed out that the effect of punishment is dependent on its timing. If punishment occurs before reward the act will tend to be inhibited, whereas if reward precedes the punishment, it will tend to be reinforced The importance of this time sequence has been demonstrated in children with social punishment (Aronfreed and Reber, 1965). Eysenck (1964) has suggested that it is the carefully arranged time sequence which distinguishes aversion therapy from 'punishment' as usually understood. Punishment is a relatively arbitrary and long-delayed consequence of an action and would therefore be expected to have little influence on the habit in question. Aversion therapy is arranged so that the aversive stimulus is given before any positive reinforcement consequent on the act is experienced. Obviously this can be very difficult to achieve in practice as split-second timing is required.

The effects of punishment are complex and often difficult to predict. As early as 1944, Estes's studies showed that responses inhibited by punishment may only be suppressed, for they may reappear in situations where punishment is weaker or absent. Punishment may in fact actually prevent the extinction of a habit if it inhibits it sufficiently to prevent its occurring without rewarding consequences. However, there is evidence that punishment can both weaken responses (Church, 1963; Solomon, 1964) and strengthen them (Greenwald, 1965). This paradoxical effect may occur when the behaviour that is punished is itself a conditioned avoidance response motivated by anxiety. Punishment may increase anxiety and therefore strengthen the avoidance response. Eysenck and Rachman (1965) suggest that aversion therapy may worsen behaviour mediated by anxiety. The patient who drinks to reduce his anxiety may also drink to reduce the anxiety and pain evoked by punishment. In keeping with this, Beech (1960) showed that aversion therapy can worsen writer's cramp in highly anxious subjects.

It appears that the nature, intensity and timing of aversive stimuli, together with the subjects' anxiety level and previous experience of punishment, are important variables in determining the consequences of punishment. Severe punishment can lead to disorganization of behaviour and maladaptive responses. As a result of these consider-ations, more attention is given to the development of new adaptive responses to replace the maladaptive. Raymond (1964) introduced a choice situation during the aversion treatment of alcoholics. Without prior warning or explanation, a patient is given an injection of saline instead of apomorphine which has been given in the previous sessions. In the treatment room there is a selection of soft drinks in addition to alcoholic ones. When the patient chooses a soft drink (which invari-ably he does) the therapist encourages the patient and assures him that he will not experience any nausea or vomiting. The operant response of the patient selecting a soft drink is rewarded by the relaxation in atmosphere and the omission of the aversive stimulus.

A similar rationale underlies the techniques of aversion relief therapy described by Thorpe *et al.* (1964b). These authors used verbal cues in the treatment of homosexuals. The patient has to read aloud a series of words as they appear on a screen and receives a shock as he does so. The last word is a 'relief' word such as 'heterosexual' for which no shock is given. If the patient fails to read out the non-relief words he is given a more intense shock. Feldman rightly criticizes this part of the technique, because the patient is 'punished' for not reading aloud a previously attractive word, and this would be expected to strengthen the response rather than eliminate it.

Wilde (1964) incorporated a relief stimulus in his treatment of cigarette addiction. He used an apparatus consisting of two electric ventilators mounted on a rotating disc, one delivering hot cigarette smoke into the subject's face, the other menthol flavoured air at room temperature. The patient is required to light and smoke his favourite cigarette while the aversive stimulus is administered and to continue smoking for as long as he can tolerate it. When he puts the cigarette out and says 'I want to give up smoking' the noxious air is replaced by 'refreshing' mentholated air. Several trials are given in each treatment session which is ended with the patient lighting a cigarette without receiving the aversive stimulus, in the hope that he experiences that lighting a cigarette is now devoid of pleasure.

Goldiamond (1965) has employed DAF as an aversive stimulus in which the patient is given a miniature delay instrument which is worn in a similar way to a hearing aid. The instrument has a switch which allows the subject to turn it on and off and also to adjust the amount of delay to produce the best result. An advantage of this method is that it can be used outside the consulting room.

Feldman (Feldman and MacCulloch, 1965; Feldman, 1966) has elaborated a technique of aversion therapy which attempts to make the maximum use of the known experimental findings in the field of learning. Originally the method was used in the treatment of homosexuals but recently it has been extended to other sexual deviations. Instrumental avoidance learning with electric shock as the aversive stimulus is used for the reasons already discussed. They also attempt to incorporate the following features which have been shown to increase resistance to extinction:

1. Spaced rather than massed treatment sessions.
2. Maintenance of contiguity of stimulus and response throughout treatment.
3. The strength of shock should vary randomly about the level reported by the patient to be unpleasant and should not be increased gradually.
4. Partial reinforcement should be used in which the reinforced and non-reinforced trials are randomly alternated.
5. The partial reinforcement schedule should include both variable ratio and interval schedules.
6. There should be a variable delay between the start of the undesired behaviour and the onset of the aversive stimulus.
7. The treatment situations should be both realistic and varied.

In addition to these considerations, the authors argue in favour of the use of realistic photographs because of the ease with which such stimuli can be manipulated. They also emphasize the importance of encouraging substitute adaptive responses and suggest the use of 'relief' stimuli to shape them. Finally, they make out a strong case for using graded stimulus hierarchies, starting by establishing aversion to the mildly attractive stimuli and gradually progressing to the most attractive ones. The reverse order is recommended for the 'relief' stimuli. Their treatment technique appears to meet most of the above requirements. The homosexual patient grades a series of photographic slides of men and women in order of their sexual attractiveness to him. He sits in front of the projection screen and has a switch which can remove the slide. The slides are projected in order according to the two hierarchies, starting with the least attractive man and the most attractive woman. At first the male slides are projected for eight seconds and a shock is given if the patient has not switched off the slide by then. When stable avoidance behaviour has been established, three types of trials, randomly interspersed, are introduced. The first consists of reinforced trials in which the patient's attempt to remove the slide is immediately successful. In the second type there is a varying delay between pressing the switch and removal of the slide. The third type consists of non-reinforced trials in which the patient is shocked whether or not he makes the avoidance response of switching off the slide. Furthermore, on 40 per cent of the trials, randomly selected, a female slide is projected for ten seconds as soon as the patient switches off the male slide. The patient can ask for the female slide to be returned, but his request is complied with in a random manner. The inter-trial intervals vary between fifteen and thirty-five seconds, and about twenty-five stimulus presentations are given in a twenty-minute session.

The aversion techniques described so far have been used mainly in the treatment of patients whose chief disorder is characterized by manifest abnormal behaviour. However, aversion therapy has also been applied to problems of a compulsive or ideational nature (e.g. Kushner, 1967; Wolpe, 1958). The patient can use a portable shock apparatus whenever disturbing thoughts or impulses occur. Involuntary motor movements have also been treated with aversion therapy.

Liversedge and Sylvester (1955) treated a small group of patients with writer's cramp. This condition has components of tremor and spasm. To deal with the tremor, the patients were required to insert a stylus into a series of progressively smaller holes. Whenever this made contact with the edge of the hole a circuit was completed which delivered a shock to the free hand. In the next stage of treatment, the patient had to trace straight, curved and zig-zag lines on a metal plate, and any deviation from the path resulted in a shock. To counteract the spasm the patients had to write with a special pen so designed that excessive thumb pressure on it resulted in a shock being delivered to the other hand. A similar principle has been employed in the treatment of torticollis (Brierley, 1967).

The methods of aversion therapy so far described are unpleasant and most therapists are reluctant to employ them if better forms of treatment are available. Clearly there are also ethical considerations involved which are discussed in chapter 7. To overcome some of these objections, a technique not requiring the presentation of external noxious stimuli has been elaborated. Treatment relies instead on the use of imagined or covert stimuli, which are assumed to be subject to the same laws as overt behaviour. Perhaps the first published account of this technique is that of Lazarus (1958) who suggested to a patient with a compulsive neurosis that he begin to feel anxious when imagining the performance of the compulsive act and calm when resisting the temptation to indulge in it. Gold and Neufeld (1965) included in a treatment programme imagined homosexual situations followed immediately by imagined aversive stimuli such as the presence of a policeman. A similar technique was employed by Kolvin (1967) which she called 'aversive imagery therapy'. Cautela (1966, 1967) reported several cases illustrating ingenious variations of this procedure which he named 'covert sensitization'. An alcoholic patient was trained to relax and imagine vividly both drinking alcohol with its feeling of satisfaction and the experience of nausea and vomiting with their unpleasant concomitants. In subsequent sessions the patient is relaxed and asked to signal as soon as he has imagined the sight of a drink and the desire for it, but before he picks up the glass. When the patient signals he is asked immediately to imagine nausea and vomiting. He is instructed to continue with the procedure when at home. Davison

(1968a and b) has used a slightly modified technique in the treatment of a sadist and an adolescent with a behaviour disorder.

Homme (1965) has described a 'control of coverants' technique. Coverants are covert operants such as thoughts and fantasies. The patient is taught to develop self-control by making a covert response which is incompatible with the undesired overt behaviour. A habitual smoker was encouraged to imagine a situation in which he does not feel like smoking (e.g. after having seen a film about lung cancer) whenever he felt like smoking. If successful in performing the covert response, positive reinforcement was given (e.g. a cup of coffee) in order to strengthen it.

Experience with covert techniques is limited and their range of applicability and efficacy not yet established. They have some advantages over the more conventional aversive procedures but there are also disadvantages. They appear deceptively simple but the lack of control over the relevant stimuli is a serious drawback.

Negative practice

Methods of treatment based on negative practice, sometimes referred to as exhaustion, satiation or extinction, derive from the principle that the massed practice of a learned response without reinforcement leads to its extinction.

Claims that repetitive habits such as tics could be eliminated by making the subject repeat them voluntarily were made long ago (Dunlap, 1932). Lehner (1954) reviewed the literature up to 1951 on the use of negative practice and gave a detailed account of his own use of the method. Yates (1958) has discussed the rationale of this treatment and investigated the optimal conditions for the elimination of tics in a patient with multiple tics. He adopted the two-factor theory of learning, and considered that some tics were drive-reducing, avoidance responses originally acquired in a traumatic situation. Others, particularly in children, might be acquired by imitation, or as an avoidance response to a noxious stimulus such as a tight collar. In order to account for the performance of the tic at a given moment he employs the Hullian concepts of multiplicative function of the habit strength of the tic and the momentary drive strength of anxiety.

Massed practice of the tic should lead to a build-up of reactive inhibition (RI) and extinction of the tic will result from conditioned inhibition. Furthermore, there should be no risk of increasing its habit strength, since it is already at its maximum. Successful treatment is therefore considered to be the extinction of a learned habit of maximal strength by massed, non-reinforced practice. In so far as Hull considers extinction to be due to the conditioning of the incompatible response of resting, negative practice itself could be considered another variant of counter-conditioning. However, on operational grounds, it seems legitimate to regard it as distinct. The therapist does not 'impose' an incompatible response on the patient. It is assumed to arise as a result of massed practice.

Yates's orientation was experimental rather than therapeutic and his main interest lay in determining the optimal technique for negative practice. The standard procedure adopted was a minimum of five one-minute periods of massed practice of each tic with an interval of one minute between each period. There were two sessions a day, one under supervision of the therapist and the other at home without supervision. The maximum duration of massed practice for one tic was one hour. After four sessions the patient had a three-week rest. Yates concluded that the best results were obtained by the combination of prolonged massed practice followed by prolonged rest. The tic must be reproduced as precisely and intensively as possible, and repeated to the point of exhaustion in order to build up a high level of reactive inhibition (Wolpe and Lazarus, 1966).

Rafi (1962) adopted Yates's technique in the treatment of two tiqueurs, using a two hour intensive practice session with a one-week rest interval in one case. Lazarus (1961b) describes a similar method, and Walton (1961, 1964) has given chlorpromazine and amylobarbitone before the massed practice sessions, on the theoretical assumption that any reduction in anxiety achieved would decrease tolerance to reactive inhibition and so enhance conditioned inhibition.

Clark (1966) has employed negative practice in the treatment of Gilles de la Tourette's syndrome. The patient was required to repeat aloud as frequently as possible the currently favoured obscenity. One-minute practice was alternated with one-minute rest periods. An electric shock was given if different words were interpolated during the practice session or if there was any tic during the rest period. To counteract any tendency for voluntary rest pauses during the practice minute, the patient was instructed to speak the word in time with the beat of a metronome.

Methods akin to negative practice have been incorporated in the treatment of stammering. The stammerer may be required to 'fake' his stammer by deliberately repeating syllables (Meissner, 1946) or to repeat each stammered word in a passage read aloud until fluency is achieved (Sheehan, 1951; Sheehan and Voas, 1957). The latter authors considered that they were reinforcing the approach responses of fluent speech rather than the avoidance response of stammering. Case (1960) made his patients reproduce their stammer as accurately as possible and sometimes also administered electric shocks in an effort to reproduce the emotional state which was assumed to accompany their stuttering.

Other treatment techniques have been formulated in terms of reactive and conditioned inhibition and are therefore claimed to be examples of negative practice. Walton (1960) has argued that if the secondary rewards which maintain a symptom can be removed, the symptom itself will be eliminated by its unreinforced practice and resultant conditioned inhibition. He illustrated his thesis with an example of a patient with long-standing neurodermatitis and 'compulsive scratching' thought to be maintained by secondary rewards. Environmental manipulation aimed at eliminating the assumed rewards succeeded in eliminating the scratching and the rash. However, the patient was not required to carry out massed practice of his scratching (in fact this would have caused excessive skin damage), and it is therefore doubtful whether this therapeutic procedure should be called negative practice.

Flooding (implosive) therapy

The theoretical basis of the methods of treatment discussed so far has involved either the counter-conditioning of an incompatible response or the extinction of an instrumental avoidance response by massed non-reinforced practice. The term flooding was first used by Polin (1959) to describe an extinction procedure in which rats were submitted to continuous exposure to a CS but were free to perform a previously learned instrumental avoidance response. The aim of flooding or implosive therapy is the extinction of anxiety itself by non-reinforced practice. The patient is required to remain in the feared situation and experience all the anxiety engendered, and is prevented from escaping from the situation by means of any avoidance response.

There is some experimental evidence from animal studies that preventing or delaying the escape response from a conditioned anxiety-producing stimulus hastens the extinction of that response (see Lomont, 1965). Different theoretical interpretations have been put forward to account for the underlying processes involved. If the avoidance response is considered to have been evoked by a conditioned anxiety stimulus possessing no intrinsic danger, prevention of the avoidance response would be expected to lead to extinction of the CS, following the usual process of discrimination in classical conditioning. As long as the avoidance response continues to occur, there can be no discrimination. Another interpretation of the extinction of anxiety in flooding procedures is in terms of conditioned inhibition of anxiety resulting from massed practice. If a cognitive theory of extinction is adopted, flooding is explained in terms of a change in expectancy when the subject experiences that a particular conditioned anxiety stimulus does not cause danger. Beneficial reality-testing has occurred.

Stampfl and his colleagues, in a series of papers (see Stampfl and Levis, 1967, 1968), have outlined a method of implosive therapy together with a theoretical formulation for its basis. He adopts a two-factor learning theory view of neurotic symptoms as conditioned anxiety and avoidance responses arising originally from primary noxious stimuli, but also emphasizes the importance of internal events such as thoughts and impulses which become secondarily conditioned and thereafter serve as anxiety-evoking cues.

Implosive therapy therefore starts with diagnostic interviews aimed at ascertaining both the external and internal cues which evoke overt and covert avoidance responses. An avoidance serial cue hierarchy (ASCH) is constructed. Low in the hierarchy are the anxiety cues of which the subject is most aware and which usually cause symptoms. Higher in the hierarchy are the sequential cues thought to be more closely related to the primary aversive stimulus. These cues may only become apparent during treatment, and tend to include 'psycho-dynamic-type' cues such as aggressive and sexual conflicts, including castration fear and Oedipal wishes.

Treatment consists of having the patient imagine the feared situation as vividly as possible and experience all the emotion that this elicits. The therapist's aim is to maintain the patient's anxiety at as high a level as possible, which is done by describing progressively more fearful scenes to be imagined, including the sequential cues which the therapist suspects are involved. Low-item hierarchy cues are presented first, and only when the patient's anxiety level starts to fall are higher items introduced. Individual sessions last for about thirty to sixty minutes, and are arranged so that they end at a time when anxiety is reduced. After several such sessions with the therapist, the patient is instructed to re-enact the scenes himself until anxiety is reduced.

Implosive therapy invites comparison with Wolpe's systematic desensitization, for both involve exposing the patient to his anxiety-evoking situations. But in systematic desensitization inhibition of anxiety is required so that an antagonistic response can occur, whereas implosive therapy requires maximum experience of anxiety to enable it to be extinguished. Stampfl adopts some Freudian concepts of internal conflicts, but pleads that this need not lead to outright rejection of internal cues in treatment, because these are valid at an operational level if they do in fact evoke anxiety (Stampfl and Levis, 1968).

There have been few published reports of implosive treatment. Hogan (1966) gives an account of short-term treatment of psychotic patients. Hogan and Kirchner (1967) treated twenty-one volunteer co-ed students who were phobic of rats with one session of implosive therapy lasting thirty to forty minutes, and Levis and Carrera (1967) treated ten neurotic out-patients with ten implosive sessions of about an hour each.

Malleson (1959) employed a similar method in treating a student with 'examination panic' by making him imagine intensely disturbing examination situations without being relaxed. The exposure trials were massed. The author also briefly states that he employed a similar technique with agoraphobic patients. Wolpin and Raines (1966) treated two patients with a fear of snakes by asking them to imagine for a period of ten minutes the most disturbing items in the fear hierarchy. Meyer (1966) describes the treatment of two patients with compulsive rituals. They were persuaded to make contact with or handle the actual objects which evoked anxiety and the compulsive rituals, but were prevented from carrying out the rituals. A variety of methods were employed to achieve this, including encouragement, distraction, supervision and separation from objects required in the performance of the ritual (e.g. wash-bas n). Meyer conceptualized his treatment in cognitive terms such as modification of expectancies or reality testing and did not refer to this procedure as flooding.

Operant conditioning

This therapeutic method has its origin in Skinner's system of operant conditioning (Skinner, 1938). Such behaviour can be modified by the use of positive and negative reinforcement, and new patterns of response established by shaping and discrimination learning (see chapter 2). Initially Skinner's orientation was predominantly experimental and involved laboratory experiments with rats and pigeons. More recently, mainly through the work of Lindsley (e.g. Lindsley and Skinner, 1954; Lindsley, 1956, 1960), the methodology of operant conditioning has been successfully adapted to the study of human behaviour. Attention was first directed to determining the types of behaviour which could be brought under experimental control, and the types of responses which could be shaped when there was a behaviour deficit. The behaviour of psychotic and mentally subnormal patients was the first to be studied. Recently, however, this research has had increasing impact on therapists, so that operant techniques are now being applied to the study and treatment of a wider range of psychiatric disorders.

The most prominent feature of the Skinnerian approach is the tendency to focus on a specific observable symptom – the 'target behaviour'–and the environmental events which follow the behaviour, reinforce it and maintain it. Therapeutic intervention involves the manipulation of reinforcements so that the behaviour is extinguished and replaced by more adaptive responses. Reinforcement is given when desired responses are made, and withheld when there are undesired responses ('time out'). When the appropriate behaviour is lacking, successive approximations to the required response are reinforced until the new response is established. Although the concentration is on overt behaviour rather than 'inner mental states', verbal behaviour and covert responses are considered to be controlled in the same way.

Numerous illustrations of the application of operant conditioning to psychiatric patients are available in the literature (e.g. Sidman, 1962; Bachrach, 1964; Eysenck, 1964; Ullmann and Krasner, 1965; Lovaas, 1966; Davison, 1969).

It is relatively easy to see how treatment techniques are guided by the operant conditioning model, and indeed they often appear deceptively straightforward and naïve. However, the design and execution of a therapeutic programme may involve a great variety of procedures and operations, requiring considerable ingenuity in their construction. It is impossible within the scope of this book to describe all the procedures that have been employed. We give examples of methods used in the treatment of some schizophrenic behaviour, including delusions, mutism and thought disorder; some neurotic and habit disorders, and organic mental disorders.

In a series of studies, Ayllon and his colleagues have demonstrated that operant techniques can be used to modify maladaptive or socially disruptive behaviour of schizophrenic hospital patients in closed wards (Ayllon and Michael, 1959; Ayllon and Haughton, 1962; Ayllon, 1963). They noticed that undesirable behaviour, such as excessive washing or floor scrubbing, hoarding and feeding disturbances, was being socially reinforced by the nursing staff when they gave extra attention to those patients exhibiting the disturbed behaviour. The nurses were instructed to give or withhold reinforcement according to the patient's behaviour. Desirable behaviour was rewarded by attention, conversation, food and cigarettes. In other words, undesirable behaviour was greeted with disapproval, whereas healthy behaviour was praised. Patients who usually had to be persuaded to go into the dining-room for meals were not allowed to go in late. In these procedures the patients were not told in advance the change in behaviour which was required. A later study (Ayllon and Azrin, 1964) carried out to evaluate the relative contributions of verbal instructions and positive reinforcement in training schizophrenic and mental defective patients to pick up their cutlery before entering the cafeteria, demonstrated that a combination of the procedures was the most effective.

Verbal behaviour can also be significantly altered by contingent administration of reinforcers (see Greenspoon, 1962; Williams, 1964). The frequency of coherent talk in three schizophrenics increased and babbling talk decreased when coherent talk was socially reinforced (Ayllon and Haughton, 1964). The frequency of delusional utterances of three paranoid schizophrenics was diminished as a result of the therapist and nurses strongly disagreeing with the delusional statements while positively reinforcing reality-based remarks (Kennedy, 1964). In all the studies described above, improvement in target behaviour appeared to be accompanied by more widespread beneficial effects.

A greater therapeutic challenge is presented by patients with more severe disturbances in which the desired responses are not already in their behavioural repertoire and who are not responsive to social reinforcement. An impressive example of shaping new behaviour in such a situation is provided by Peters and Jenkins's (1954) study of severely regressed chronic schizophrenics. Feeding was chosen as a primary reinforcer while the patients were inaccessible to social reinforcement. Hunger was stimulated by small doses of insulin and the patients were encouraged to take part in increasingly complex problem tasks such as simple mazes, multiple-choice learning and verbal reasoning. Fudge was given as the positive reward. After several weeks of these sessions, the insulin injections were discontinued and social rewards, which by now were more effective than food, were made contingent on solving relevant interpersonal problems which hampered the patients in their everyday life.

A similar example of shaping behaviour is provided by Isaacs et al. (1960) in their attempt to reinstate speech in two adult mute catatonic schizophrenics. The sight of chewing gum caused a momentary alteration in one patient's impassive staring expression. Chewing gum was therefore used as the reward for any eye movement, and subsequently made contingent upon facial movements, lip movements, vocalization, and finally on spoken words. At the same time the therapist urged the patient to say words.

When the desired target behaviour occurs so infrequently that re-inforcement alone is ineffective, modelling procedures have been incorporated. For example, Sherman (1965) employed imitative responses to establish shaping in chronic mute patients. One patient was rewarded initially for imitating the therapist's non-verbal behaviour such as standing up, then kissing, and finally speech of increasing complexity. The technique of 'fading' can be used to bring the desired response under more appropriate discriminative stimulus control; for example, once the patient's responses are brought under imitative control (e.g. the patient repeating the word 'horse' spoken by the therapist), the next step is to shift the control to the appropriate stimuli (the patient says 'horse' when shown a picture of a horse). The shift to naming is achieved by fading out the imitative prompts in gradual steps. In this manner words will acquire appropriate meaning.

Operant techniques are being employed increasingly frequently in the treatment of childhood psychosis. Here, autistic and destructive behaviour can be modified and attempts made to shape cognitive and social behaviour. Responsiveness and obedience in a play situation were shaped using food as reward, and secondary rewards introduced later (Davison, 1964). Echolalia was eliminated and replaced by normal speech by a combination of techniques. Initially shaping and imitation were used to develop speech, then backing of verbal prompts was introduced in order to transfer speech from imitative control to meaningful cues. 'Time out' from reinforcement was used to eliminate inappropriate behaviour, while appropriate responses were initiated and developed by differential reinforcement with food (Risley and Wolf, 1967).

A more complex programme was employed by Lovaas (1966) in an experimental ward with six mute autistic children who present a more difficult problem as they have no speech at all initially. Food is given first to reward any sounds uttered, and then only for sounds uttered immediately after the therapist has made a sound. Subsequently the child has to repeat the same sound as the therapist to obtain reinforcement. In the next stage two sounds have to be imitated and discrimination between them is established. Gradually the child learns to imitate any sound made by the therapist. Finally the imitative stimuli are replaced by more appropriate stimuli for particular words so that they are used meaningfully. Leff (1968) has reviewed the operant conditioning techniques used in the treatment of childhood psychosis. More recently a similar method for training autistic children has been described by Martin *et al.* (1968) for problem behaviour, speech, tracing and matching, in which they emphasize the withholding of any potentially reinforcing response by the therapist to the child's inattentive or undesirable behaviour. They also extended individual treatment into a classroom situation.

A somewhat different application of operant treatment has been employed in the everyday management of a ward of adult schizophrenic patients. Much interest has been shown in the 'token economy' system developed by Ayllon and Azrin (1965, 1968). They employed Premack's principle, which states that for any pair of responses which can occur in a given situation, the one that has a greater probability of taking place will function as a reinforcer for the less probable one (Premack, 1959). Reinforcing activities such as sitting in the day-room, watching television and obtaining certain privileges were made contingent on desired behaviour such as walking, dressing tidily, making beds and attending the workshop. To bridge the gap between the performance of the target behaviour and the presumed reinforcing effect of higher probability responses, Ayllon and Azrin introduced tokens which were given to the patients immediately after they had performed the target behaviour. The tokens could be used later to obtain the privilege to engage in the higher probability behaviour of watching television, etc. This programme was implemented by the nursing staff both with patients unable to leave the ward and with patients who were already able to engage in activities outside the ward. Controlled studies showed that tokens given to reward desirable behaviour increased its frequency. Removal or random administration of tokens led to a decrease in the frequency of target behaviour.

Similar 'token economy' systems designed to promote behaviour which would contribute to satisfactory adjustment outside the hospital have now been reported (e.g. Gericke, 1965; Atthowe and Krasner, 1968). Modification of treatment as progress occurred included delaying of reinforcement, with tokens given weekly and finally allowing patients to buy themselves out of the system by obtaining a *carte blanche* which served instead of tokens. A recent review of token economy programmes has been published by Krasner (1968).

115

In hospital, the patients themselves can take part in the management of the ward (Fairweather, 1964). They can make collective decisions regarding job assignments, personal problems and the allocation of rewards such as money and passes. Responsible behaviour led to increasing rewards and promotion. In order to encourage collective responsibility and the active participation of every patient, the group itself was rewarded with promotions for making sound recommendations. The group also planned the discharge and subsequent employment of their members.

There are numerous reports of the treatment of neurotic and conduct disorders in children. Thumb-sucking was decreased by interrupting a film cartoon the child was watching each time he sucked his thumb (Baer, 1962). Encopresis has been treated by taking the child to the lavatory after each meal and at bedtime. If he appeared anxious in the lavatory, he was given a sweet to suck or a comic to read. If defecation was painful as a result of constipation, a bulk laxative was given. If there was no bowel movement, no reward or punishment was given, but if defecation did occur, the child was rewarded with food and praise. The rewards were changed according to the child's current interests as the efficacy of a particular reward decreased. Once the child became accustomed to using the lavatory and had stopped soiling himself, he was instructed to go to the lavatory whenever he felt the urge to defecate. Rewards were given when he reported successful defecation (Neal, 1963).

Operant techniques have been carried out by therapists, nursing staff and patients. Obviously, it is logical to extend this to include parents and teachers who may be providing reinforcement contingencies which maintain behaviour disturbances such as temper tantrums, hyperactivity, and overdependency (e.g. Russo, 1964; Straugham, 1964; Whaler *et al.*, 1965; Hawkins, *et al.*, 1966; O'Leary *et al.*, 1967). A detailed functional analysis is made of the occurrence and pattern of the behaviour, and the response of the parents and teacher. This assessment may be conducted at home or in a playroom. As a result of this, the therapist may be able to show the parent how to change his responses to the child so that the deviant behaviour is unrewarded and desirable behaviour rewarded. A mother who has tended to pay extra attention to the child when he has a temper tantrum, and little attention when he plays constructively, is instructed to reverse her behaviour so that the constructive behaviour is rewarded. Primary or social rewards and tokens can be employed (e.g. O'Leary *et al.*, 1967). School phobias have been treated by a combination of operant reinforcement to establish attendance at school and systematic desensitization to reduce the anxieties evoked by the school situation (e.g. Lazarus *et al.*, 1965; Patterson, 1965). Relaxation, reassurance and gradual intro- duction to the school situation was followed by positive reinforcement with comics or tokens for achieving the successive stages in school attendance.

Operant techniques have not often been used as the sole method of treatment of neurotic disorders in adults. Bachrach *et al.* (1965) treated a patient with severe anorexia nervosa by restricting initially most comforts and conversation and using them as positive rewards for eating. Gradually as eating became established and weight gained, social rewards and privileges were given. Barrett (1962) reduced the frequency of multiple tics in a patient by having him listen to music which was interrupted every time a tic occurred. This proved to be more effective than self-control or continuous music or tic-produced white noise. There was some reduction in the tic rate between treat- ment sessions.

Some patients with hysterical perceptual disturbances have been treated by conditioning methods which demonstrate to the patient that normal perception can occur. An operant conditioning technique applied to hysterical blindness by Brady and Lind (1961) involved positive reward of praise and privileges when he pressed a button at eighteen- to twenty-one-second intervals, and disapproval when his timing was poor. A buzzer was sounded whenever the pressing was correctly timed. After several sessions a light bulb was switched on to indicate the correct time for pressing without the patient being in- formed. There was no improvement in performance and he appeared anxious. However, when he was told that the light would help him to time his button pressing correctly, his performance improved. After twenty-six such treatment sessions he again became anxious but announced that he could see. Eventually he was able to make fine visual discriminations in treatment sessions and could also see outside the treatment session. This patient relapsed after several months and was reinvestigated by Zimmerman and Grosz (1966). They were able to bring operant responses under the control of visual cues again but also demonstrated the significant effect of social approval. In the final treatment session the patient was praised for performing 'like a blind person' and criticized for responding as a person with normal sight would. The patient's performance was influenced by this procedure and he continued to behave as if he were blind.

The above procedures suggest that making the patient consciously aware of perception could be a useful therapeutic procedure. Other conditioning techniques have been employed for this purpose (e.g. Hilgard and Marquis, 1940; Malmo *et al.*, 1952). Hilgard and Marquis treated a patient with an hysterical anaesthesia and paralysis of one arm. Initially, electric shock was applied repeatedly to the normal hand as the UCS for finger withdrawal, preceded by the CS of similar shocks delivered to the anaesthetic hand. Sensation in this hand returned gradually. After this, very weak shocks were applied to the normal hand followed by strong shocks to the abnormal hand. Conditioned withdrawal movements appeared in the affected hand.

In concluding this account of some behaviour therapy techniques, mention of their application to problems outside the usual range of psychiatric disorders will be made. Educational backwardness and poor reading ability of retarded, emotionally disturbed and culturally deprived children have been improved by the use of tokens and bonuses as positive rewards for correct reading and answers (Staats *et al.*, 1967).

Symptoms which, in part at least, are consequent on brain damage, may also be subjected to operant control. Efron (1957) described an epileptic patient whose temporal lobe fits could be arrested by a scent presented during the aura. By pairing the sight of a bracelet with the scent, the bracelet alone acquired the ability to evoke the odour and terminate the fit. At a later stage, 'thinking about the bracelet' could arrest the fit, and finally it appeared that spontaneous inhibition of fits coincided with an 'hallucination' of the specific scent used in the treatment.

The hyperactive behaviour of a brain-damaged boy was diminished initially by pairing an auditory stimulus with positive reinforcement (sweets and money) for every ten-second period in which the boy was attentive. After this the auditory stimulus alone was used as the reward for attending in the classroom, and tangible rewards were given after the lessons (Patterson *et al.*, 1965).

As a final example of the application of behaviour therapy, Macpherson's (1967) treatment of the involuntary movements of a patient with Huntington's chorea will be cited. At first intensive training in relaxation was given. As voluntary movement of one part of the body had tended to trigger off involuntary movements in another part, the patient was then trained to relax while carrying out voluntary movements. In the next stage of treatment the patient was taught to perceive the sensations associated with the start of an involuntary movement by amplification through headphones of the electromyographic tracing from the affected muscle through an audiometer. The onset of muscle contraction was therefore signalled through the headphone to the patient so that she could learn to recognize the afferent sensations arising from the limb at the start of an involuntary contraction. Finally the patient was taught to relax the muscles involved as soon as the first sensation of contraction was perceived.

Conclusions

This review of the main treatment methods used in behaviour therapy demonstrates a multiplicity of techniques which are continuing to proliferate. Such diversity is of itself disconcerting, and confusion is added by differences in terminology and failure to distinguish between operational description of methods and their supposed theoretical basis. It is hardly surprising that this has led to an undesirable rift between learning theorists and behaviour therapists (see Rachman and Eysenck, 1966, and Wilson and Evans, 1967, for a more extensive discussion of some of these issues).

It is frequently stated that in so far as 'modern learning theory' does not exist, behaviour therapy techniques cannot be said to be derived from it. No one would claim that there is a single coherent theory of learning which accounts for human behaviour. There is insufficient agreement on many theoretical points to allow testable predictions to be made and therapeutic techniques to be constructed (e.g. Breger and

McGaugh, 1965). However, there is general agreement on certain well-established experimental findings concerning the relationships between classes of variables. Controversy centres around the theoretical interpretation of these findings. The same phenomena may be conceptualized in terms of Hullian, Skinnerian or Tolmanian concepts according to inclination, while the method of treatment adopted is fashioned on accepted experimental findings. In practice the same technique may be adopted whether a cognitive or an s–r reinforcement theory is favoured.

The plethora of techniques available, their mutual independence, and the derivation of different methods from the same theory or similar methods from different theories would appear to support the criticism that it is difficult to see any connexion between the behaviour methods and learning principles (see Kiesler, 1966). But this seems to be an overstatement if one accepts the distinction drawn above between experimental findings and theoretical interpretation. Unfortunately, behaviour therapists have themselves contributed to this confusion by using different terms for similar procedures and failing to separate descriptive and theoretical terms. For example, the term 'negative practice' was introduced as an operational description of a particular method of treatment. However, it has also been referred to in terms such as extinction, conditioned inhibition and reactive inhibition. Extinction is itself a descriptive term for the reduction or elimination of a response by non-reinforced practice, while the other two terms are hypothetical constructs of a particular theory of extinction. Similarly, 'systematic desensitization' describes a procedure which is also sometimes described as counter-conditioning or reciprocal inhibition. These latter terms refer to assumed processes underlying systematic desensitization.

Differences between methods are often accentuated unduly. As Wilson and Evans (1967) have pointed out, the difference between extinction and desensitization lies in 'the structuring of the learning situation'. The bell and pad treatment of enuresis can just as easily be regarded as the elimination of a bad habit as the acquisition of a new habit (Eysenck, 1960a). Similarly, operant and respondent techniques should be regarded as complementary rather than as entirely separate. The recent tendency to combine several techniques in treatment makes the frequent exaggeration of differences between methods unjustified.

It is true that no routine methods of behaviour therapy involving standard procedures of administration have yet been experimentally established. 'Crucial procedural factors' are often derived from uncontrolled clinical observation and need to be submitted to experimental investigation. Some of the therapeutic strategies used by behaviour therapists were in use long before the advent of formal behaviour therapy (Breger and McGaugh, 1965). But it is fair to add that they were not employed so explicitly or systematically. Behaviour therapy is still in its infancy. Existing methods are undergoing modification and new developments can emerge as a result of rigorous analysis of experimental findings. The accumulation of further knowledge in the field of learning can be expected to lead to new advances in treatment methods.

At present the behaviour therapist is guided by principles of learning when a programme of treatment is constructed for his patients. But the actual carrying out of treatment will depend quite largely on the therapist's ingenuity and the specific requirements of individual patients. Behaviour therapy does not refer to any one specific theory or method. It is more an approach which attempts to apply the findings of experimental psychology to the modification of abnormal and undesirable behaviour.

Chapter 5

The Efficacy of Behavior Therapy

Persuasive theoretical formulations and encouraging reports of the successful treatment of individual cases do not constitute sufficient grounds for the acceptance of behaviour therapy into clinical practice. There is no substitute for sound empirical evidence concerning the efficacy of treatment and the types of disorder and patient which respond to it. Such evidence can only be gathered by controlled investigation in which the inclusion of a matched untreated control group assessed at the same points in time as the treated group should be a minimum requirement.

The clinician will want to know whether a particular method of behaviour therapy produces better results than no treatment, and if it does, how it compares with the results of other forms of treatment, whether its efficacy depends on 'non-specific' factors or specific constituents of behaviour therapy. Finally, if specific behavioural mechanisms prove to be relevant, the crucial operations upon which success is contingent need to be identified. In addition to these practical questions at an operational level, there remains the question of the validity of the theoretical basis of the treatment and its aetiological implications. These are separate questions which may or may not be related.

In this chapter we review the evidence concerning the applicability and efficacy of behaviour therapy. Identification of the critical therapeutic mechanisms and theoretical analyses are discussed in the next chapter.

Range of applicability

It is too soon to draw any firm conclusions about the types of psychiatric disorder in which behaviour therapy may be useful. In theory it should be possible to modify most symptoms, whatever their origin, by behaviour techniques. However, because of theoretical and practical considerations, they have been employed chiefly with patients who have fairly isolated symptoms elicited by definable stimuli. In conditions susceptible to analysis in terms of Hullian s–r theory, a relatively well-tried-out treatment technique is available. The treatment of phobic patients by desensitization is the best established method of behaviour therapy. It is more difficult to apply an s–r paradigm when symptoms are diffuse, pervasive or fluctuating and their eliciting stimuli are obscure. Many personality disorders and neuroses, as well as the psychoses, fall into this category. Nevertheless, attempts to apply behaviour therapy techniques have been made in almost the whole range of psychiatric disorder.

A few generalizations derived from theoretical considerations and clinical experience have been made about the applicability of the commonly used techniques. Systematic desensitization is most effective in disorders mediated by anxiety, but is of little value in developing new adaptive habits. Operant techniques are more promising in this respect, as is the positive conditioning treatment of enuresis. Aversion therapy is used mainly for the elimination of pleasurable but maladaptive behaviour such as addictions and sexual deviations when alternative, more adaptive responses are available to the patient. Systematic desensitization and aversion techniques are less appropriate for children, in whom operant conditioning is both easy to apply and often effective.

Although these indications are based on some theoretical and clinical evidence, an uncritical and rigid adherence to them would lead to the misapplication of behaviour therapy. The choice of treatment rests ultimately on a careful analysis of the problems and requirements of each patient rather than the specific diagnosis. Even the most fanatic Skinnerian, interpreting systematic desensitization in operant terms, would admit that the elimination of a severe phobia by operant conditioning alone would be extremely difficult, if not impossible. Behaviour therapists are gradually becoming aware of the limitations of rigidly applying particular therapeutic techniques according to the diagnostic label and it is becoming more common to employ a combination of methods. At the present time behaviour therapy may play a significant role in the treatment of phobic anxiety states, alcoholism, sexual deviations, stammering, tics and enuresis. They have at times been successfully employed in psychoses, psychosomatic disorders, obsessional neuroses and childhood behaviour disorders. In many of these, behaviour therapy will form one part of the programme of management and will be combined with other forms of treatment.

Efficacy of behaviour therapy

Any claims made on behalf of treatment must be assessed against the natural history of the disorder or its 'spontaneous remission' rate (see Eysenck, 1960a, 1963b; Eysenck and Rachman, 1965). Unfortunately, the evidence concerning the 'spontaneous' recovery rate for various disorders is not very clear and there is considerable controversy about the accuracy of quoted figures. In his well-known review, Eysenck (1960b) concluded that about two-thirds of severe neurotics improve considerably or recover within two years without systematic psychotherapy and he suggested that 'any therapeutic method must show appreciably better results than this if it is to be taken seriously'.

Many workers have seriously questioned this conclusion (see Kiesler, 1966). It is accepted that a significant proportion of patients with the diagnosis 'neurotic illness' improve or recover within a year, with or without psychiatric treatment. However, there is a wide range of variation in the duration of neurotic disorders which is related to the type of illness and personality of the patient. As a result of this it is virtually meaningless to state the prognosis of an unselected sample of patients who only have in common the diagnostic label 'neurosis' or 'personality disorder'. There is evidence that a proportion of these 'minor psychiatric disorders' run an extremely chronic course and are responsible to some extent for the increasing prevalence of psychiatric illness with age (Shepherd *et al.*, 1966). Some neurotic disorders such as the obsessional states and many of the personality disorders have a worse prognosis than the over-all figure of 70 per cent remission would lead one to expect. This is well illustrated by the results of some of the clinical trials which are discussed in the following chapters. Eysenck's conclusions were based on two studies.

The first was an American survey conducted by Landis (1937) who reported that 70 per cent of 'neurotic' patients admitted to hospital were discharged within a year. The second was Denker's (1947) study of 500 American insurance disability claimants with neurotic disorders, 72 per cent of whom 'recovered' in two years. But hospitalized patients and insurance claimants hardly form a sample comparable to the neurotic patients referred to the psychiatrist. Hospitalized patients are likely to have been more severely ill, and insurance claimants less ill. However, the main point is that any sample of patients included under the heading 'neurosis' is likely to be so heterogeneous that little useful information can be obtained. In considering prognosis, type, duration and severity of the neurotic disorder are important variables. In addition, the patients in both the studies quoted received some treatment, if not interpretative psychotherapy. Indeed, it is difficult for patients not to receive some form of therapy (see Goldstein, 1960). Finally, the method of assessment of recovery was dissimilar in the two studies and unlike the usual methods adopted in assessing the effects of psychotherapy. Recent reviews of psychological treatment, emphasizing both its therapeutic effect and its sometimes deleterious effect or absence of effect, have been published by Bergin (1967) and Kellner (1967).

There is little doubt that remissions can occur in neurotic disorders without professional psychiatric treatment, and that this occurs more frequently in some types of neurosis than in others. Several theoretical explanations have been put forward to account for this. Learning theorists would expect some changes in symptomatology to occur as a result of learning processes occurring haphazardly, some of which may be therapeutic. Wolpe (1958) considered that the principle of reciprocal inhibition would account for some spontaneous recovery because responses antagonistic to anxiety could occur by chance in the ordinary course of life at a point in time when they would lead to the reciprocal inhibition of anxiety. Eysenck (1963a) argues that, in terms of learning principles, a gradual extinction of conditioned fear responses should take place over the course of time provided that the patient has not developed total avoidance of the situation and that he encounters it without concurrent re-exposure to the original unconditioned stimulus. Eysenck considers that the time course of 'spontaneous remission' resembles a typical extinction curve.

These two theoretical explanations of remission in terms of reciprocal inhibition or extinction of conditioned avoidance responses are not incompatible because both include the concept of inhibition to account for extinction. But they appear only to offer an explanation for neurotic behaviour mediated by anxiety, which Eysenck calls 'unadaptive surplus response-habits'. Yet patients with 'surplus habits' are characterized by strong and persistent avoidance behaviour, so it seems unlikely that they should have such a high 'spontaneous remission' rate as 70 per cent.

In psychiatric disorders which are thought to be due to a failure to learn adaptive responses (e.g. childhood enuresis, encopresis, ephemia), 'spontaneous remission' involves successful learning. Rachman (1963) has suggested that sudden or rapid improvement following a new incentive, particularly if the patient has been exposed previously to the learning situation without success, is due to latent learning. This phenomenon can be demonstrated experimentally, when sudden and large increments in performance occur when appropriate reinforcement is given after a period of practice without obvious reinforcement.

Clearly it is possible to explain the phenomenon of 'spontaneous remission' of some disorders in terms of learning principles. However, it would be a formidable task to test the validity of these theories when so many chance factors are invoked. Explanation in learning terms of 'spontaneous recovery' in disorders such as depression and schizophrenia has not yet been offered. Relevant factors would include the conceptual aetiological framework employed, the importance of environmental factors, and the interaction of the patient with relatives and friends.

Unfortunately, there is also a scarcity of sound critical evidence regarding the results of specific therapeutic methods. Several reports of treatment of large series of patients are subject to damaging criticism (see Breger and McGaugh, 1965). Most of them have not dealt adequately with the methodological problems. Sampling biases are common. Assessment of improvement is often made only by the therapist who conducted treatment or others subject to particular observer bias. The reliability of ratings is frequently not reported. Patients who have not completed a certain number of treatment sessions may be excluded from the results. When several therapeutic methods have been used together there has seldom been sufficient experimental control exercised to assess the effect of a particular technique. Frequently no adequate follow-up study has been reported and satisfactory control groups have not been used. Infrequent assessment of progress may be misleading on account of the fluctuating nature of many clinical disorders.

An additional problem arises from the difficulty in making valid comparisons between different published results of treatment. The samples of patients usually differ in the type, duration and severity of symptoms treated, and in the number and nature of other symptoms present. Furthermore, there are often differences in the detailed administration of treatment and assessment. Obviously the methodological and practical difficulties involved in assessing the treatment of patients with psychiatric disorders are immense, and one must bear them in mind when evaluating results (see Gottschalk and Auerbach, 1966).

We have not attempted a comprehensive review of the results of behaviour therapy, but have selected studies which include some control subjects and uncontrolled studies where the samples are large and relevant information is provided.

Wolpe (1958) was the first to report a systematic investigation of behaviour therapy in adult neuroses. He has been a pioneer in the field of behaviour therapy, but it is difficult to assess his results accurately. His sample was composed of 210 adults, the majority of whom were suffering from phobic and anxiety states, seen as outpatients in private practice. Systematic desensitization was the main treatment but other techniques such as assertive therapy and sexual responses were sometimes employed. Duration of treatment averaged about ten months. On a four-point scale ranging from 'cured' to 'unimproved' covering the five areas of symptoms, productivity, interpersonal relationships, sexual adjustment and vulnerability to stress, Wolpe rated approximately 90 per cent of his patients as apparently cured or much improved. One must be cautious in evaluating this remarkably good outcome because this study is subject to most of the criticisms discussed above. In particular the figure of 90 per cent does not take account of patients who dropped out of treatment, and no systematic follow-up assessment is reported.

Wolpe (1961) has given more detailed results of systematic desensitization in thirty-nine patients selected randomly from the total number of patients treated personally by this method. The thirty-nine patients are described as having sixty-eight 'phobias and allied neurotic habits'. This term appears to include a variety of interpersonal, social and sexual anxieties. Thirty-five patients (90 per cent) responded to treatment and sixty-two out of sixty-eight (91 per cent) neurotic habits were 'overcome or markedly improved'. Four patients failed to respond and six hierarchies remained unimproved. The median number of treatment sessions was 10, and the mean number of sessions per hierarchy 11·2. A follow-up study of twenty of the successfully treated patients from six months to four years after the end of treatment revealed no relapses or emergence of new symptoms. Although more information is provided in this study it is still very difficult to draw any definite conclusions from it.

Another large uncontrolled series of 408 patients treated mainly by systematic desensitization has been reported by Lazarus (1963). Other behavioural techniques of treatment were sometimes used, including assertive training, role playing, anxiety relief, negative practice and autohypnosis. Drugs were prescribed for some patients. In addition, some patients tended to abreact during ordinary interviews and 'at judicious intervals patients' revelations were interpreted in a manner which endeavoured to clarify irrationalities in their behaviour patterns and to correct misconceptions in general'. Two therapists treated each patient, and diagnostic interviews often included a number of tests and inventories. The initial severity of symptoms and areas of maladjustment were rated on a five-point scale and progress was assessed on reports from the patient and, whenever possible, an informant. Therapeutic changes were rated in a similar manner to Wolpe's, but Lazarus appears to have employed more stringent criteria of improvement. Seventy-eight per cent of the total sample showed significant improvement. Lazarus then provided a more detailed analysis of the results obtained with 126 patients with 'severe and widespread neurosis'. Excluded from the sample were patients under fifteen years of age, those with monosymptomatic disturbances, and patients who remained in treatment for less than six sessions irrespective of outcome.

In these 126 'difficult' cases, 62 per cent were rated as markedly improved or recovered after an average of fourteen sessions. Patients in the less improved or unimproved categories tended to have been rated more neurotic and introverted on pre-treatment testing. Patients with pervasive anxiety and panic attacks responded less well to treatment. Poor motivation or rapport accounted for fifteen of forty-eight failures, four were subsequently diagnosed as 'psychotic', twenty-six were considered 'intractable' and three failures were of undetermined origin. Of twenty patients followed up after an average of two years, one had relapsed, and 'very tenuous evidence' of symptom substitution was found in two cases. Lazarus' investigation suffers from as many flaws as Wolpe's, but it should be noted that a lower over-all success rate was obtained, probably because of the more stringent criteria employed, and 'difficult' cases respond less well than simple ones.

A few other uncontrolled studies can be mentioned briefly. Hussain (1964) reported a success rate of over 90 per cent in a series of 105 patients treated by 'reciprocal inhibition and reconditioning'. Little information is provided but it appears doubtful whether the treatment methods merit this description. Hypnosis seems to have been employed to give direct suggestion rather than as a means of inducing relaxation and desensitization. Schmidt *et al.* (1965) reported a 75 per cent success rate in the treatment of forty-two consecutive neurotic patients, twenty-one of whom had sexual disorders. However, this success rate did not take into account ten patients who did not complete treatment. Their findings in regard to prognostic factors were similar to those of Lazarus.

Meyer and Crisp (1966) described the results of treatment with a variety of behaviour methods in a series of fifty-four patients with 'neurotic disorders', including eleven stammerers. Twenty-eight were in-patients. At the end of treatment (a mean of twenty-five sessions with a range from three to sixty), 28 per cent patients were much improved and 44 per cent slightly improved. Of forty-nine patients followed up for a mean period of twelve months, two had relapsed.

Hain *et al.* (1966) treated twenty-seven neurotic patients, suffering from anxiety and phobic symptoms, with systematic desensitization, but 'necessarily and sometimes voluntarily' other psychotherapeutic procedures were also used. The patients were rated on a variety of scales by the therapists and an independent judge. 78 per cent showed symptomatic improvement, and 70 per cent marked general improvement after an average of nineteen sessions. Follow-up information on fourteen patients after a mean of one year revealed that of those who had shown improvement during therapy, 20 per cent had improved further, 47 per cent maintained their improvement, 20 per cent were slightly worse and 13 per cent had relapsed completely.

Friedman (1966a), using desensitization with relaxation induced by sub-anaesthetic doses of methohexitone sodium, claimed a 100 per cent success in an average of twelve sessions with twenty-five adult out-patients with 'phobic symptoms'. At follow-up (mean duration 10·5 months), 75 per cent were assessed as being much improved or recovered (Friedman and Silverstone, 1967).

With phobic children, Lazarus and Abramovitz (1962) employed emotive imagery as an anxiety-inhibiting response and obtained recovery in seven out of nine in a mean of 3·3 sessions. No relapses or symptom substitution were found on follow-up inquiry a year later. Lazarus (1959) treated eighteen phobic children with systematic desensitization based on relaxation, feeding responses, drugs and conditioned avoidance responses. All cases had improved or recovered at the end of treatment (mean of 9·4 sessions) and on follow-up at six to thirty months.

Obviously, it is not possible to draw firm conclusions from these uncontrolled studies. However, it would be difficult to avoid acquiring at least a cautious optimism about desensitization after reading about success rates ranging from 62 per cent to 100 per cent. It is therefore important to consider evidence provided by controlled trials. Early attempts to provide such evidence came from retrospective studies of behaviour therapy in neurotic disorders with matched controls at the Maudsley Hospital (Cooper, 1963; Cooper, Gelder and Marks, 1965). Twenty-nine agoraphobics (mainly in-patients) and twelve 'other phobics' were treated by practical retraining. Twelve patients received systematic desensitization in imagination in addition. Ten in-patients with obsessional rituals received both methods of treatment. Both behaviour therapy and control groups also received other forms of treatment including supportive psychotherapy and drugs. Two independent judges examined the case notes to make an assessment of the patient before, and at the end of treatment, and one month, and one year after treatment. At the end of treatment 69 per cent of agoraphobics treated with behaviour therapy had improved symptomatically and at one year the figure was 72 per cent. The respective figures for the control group were 55 per cent and 60 per cent. For other phobias there was a 100 per cent initial improvement rate with behaviour therapy which dropped to 67 per cent at a year. This compares with control figures of 27 per cent and 45 per cent. Thus patients with other phobias fared significantly better than controls at the end of treatment, but at one year some had relapsed and their superiority was no longer significant. The duration of treatment of 'other phobias' was four months for behaviour therapy and nine months for the controls. Agoraphobics who received behaviour therapy improved only slightly more than their matched controls and they received more treatment. Of the obsessional patients, 30 per cent of the behaviour therapy group and 44 per cent of the control group were improved at the end of treatment. At one year the figures were 33 per cent and 55 per cent respectively. The authors concluded that behaviour therapy was not less effective than other methods of treatment, and was definitely more effective in monosymptomatic phobias. One would agree with this cautious opinion. The results are strikingly different to those reported by Wolpe and Lazarus. However, it is only fair to point out that, apart from the usual drawbacks of retrospective studies, the sample of patients included a large proportion with severe chronic disorders. Behaviour therapy was in a very early stage of development at that time and behavioural techniques were narrow and incomplete, with the result that therapy was directed solely against the main complaint.

In a series of investigations at the Maudsley Hospital, Gelder, Marks and their colleagues have continued to study the effects of behaviour therapy. In a retrospective study Marks and Gelder (1965) reported on twenty agoraphobics and eleven animal and social phobics treated mostly by graded retraining, but some received desensitization under relaxation or hypnosis. Psychotherapy and physical treatments were also employed in some cases. Control subjects received no behaviour therapy. Most of the agoraphobics were in-patients. For agoraphobics there was no significant difference in outcome in the two groups either at the end of treatment or at a one year follow-up, improvement occurring in about 55–60 per cent. Behaviour therapy patients showed a slightly greater improvement in symptoms at the end of treatment, perhaps related to longer and more frequent treatment. On the other hand, patients with other phobias responded much better initially with behaviour therapy (100 per cent as against 30 per cent). After a year some patients had relapsed, but the behaviour therapy group still had an advantage. A few patients developed fresh symptoms, but these occurred as frequently in controls (three), as in patients receiving behaviour therapy (four). Improvement during the period of follow-up, without previous improvement during treatment, was observed in five patients in each group.

The results of the two retrospective studies discussed certainly act as a useful corrective to the unbridled optimism of the uncontrolled studies. Patients with single phobias appear to respond well to behaviour therapy, but agoraphobics are benefited much less. However, this again was a retrospective study of patients treated in the early days of behaviour therapy, and it is impossible to draw any final conclusions from this study about the value of behavioural techniques in agoraphobia. Only a proportion of the patients received systematic desensitization in imagination as opposed to gradual training *in vivo* and there is some evidence that practical retraining alone is not the most effective behaviour treatment (see chapter 6).

In three successive papers, Gelder and Marks have published the results of controlled prospective trials of behaviour therapy in phobic disorders in which a more detailed analysis of the patients and changes in their condition was undertaken. Patients were assessed by rating scales covering symptomatology and social adjustment which were completed by the therapist and an independent assessor before, during and after treatment, and at follow-up.

The first investigation (Gelder and Marks, 1966) concerned in-patient treatment of severe agoraphobia. Twenty patients, well matched on a number of relevant variables, were randomly allocated to a behaviour therapy group receiving systematic desensitization in imagination and graded retraining, or a control group receiving 'brief re-educative psychotherapy'. Both groups were seen by their therapists three times weekly for forty-five minutes. A similar proportion in each group received drug treatment in addition. Patients in behaviour therapy were also given assertive responses 'whenever appropriate'. At the end of treatment (average twenty-three weeks for behaviour therapy and nineteen weeks for control), seven out of ten in each group showed evidence of improvement in their main phobia, but much of this improvement was lost at the end of a twelve-month follow-up. In general, changes in other symptoms and social adjustment were similar in the two groups and were quite small. Only two significant improvements in social adjustment were observed at the end of treatment, work adjustment in the behaviour therapy group and interpersonal relationships outside the family in the control group, but neither had been maintained during follow-up.

This trial shows that for severely disabled agoraphobics systematic desensitization had no dramatic effect, and at the end of follow-up patients showed considerable residual social handicap. However, it should be noted that there was a tendency for behaviour therapy to produce more symptomatic improvement in the main phobia which sometimes allowed the patient to travel to work or go shopping, and fresh symptoms did not occur more frequently in the behaviour group. No conclusions can be drawn from this study about the value of psychotherapy because the psychotherapy provided was only intended to control the 'personal contact' in behaviour therapy. On the other hand it would be only fair to comment that the trial did not explore fully the greater range of behaviour techniques now available.

In another prospective investigation, Gelder *et al.* (1967) compared the effects of behaviour therapy, individual and group analytically oriented psychotherapy in forty-two out-patients suffering from agoraphobia or other phobic disorders. They were less severely ill than the in-patient agoraphobics in the previous trial and this was reflected in the therapeutic results obtained. The method of assessment was similar to that adopted in the previous study. Sixteen patients were allocated to behaviour therapy, sixteen to group psychotherapy and ten to individual psychotherapy (shortage of psychotherapists necessitated this smaller number). Behaviour therapy included desensitization in imagination and graduated retraining in real life together with assertive training and rational discussion when appropriate. Individual psychotherapy and group therapy included interpretation of transference, and analysis of patients' thoughts and feelings in relation to past and present experiences and their relevance to present phobic symptoms. Behaviour therapy was conducted one hour weekly for an average of nine months, individual psychotherapy one hour weekly for twelve months, and group therapy one-and-a-half hours weekly for eighteen months. The three treatment groups were reasonably matched for significant clinical variables and subsidiary drug therapy. Patients were followed for two years from the start of treatment so that the mean period of follow-up for behaviour therapy was fifteen months, for individual psychotherapy twelve months and for group therapy six months.

Results showed significantly greater symptomatic improvement in the desensitization group than the others at six months. At eighteen months this trend was no longer statistically significant, but nine out of sixteen behaviour therapy patients were still rated much improved in comparison with two out of sixteen group therapy and three out of ten individual psychotherapy patients. In the assessment of social adjustment, leisure adjustment improved significantly more in the desensitization group than the others and there was a tendency towards greater improvement for this group in work adjustment. Relationships with friends improved equally with behaviour therapy and group psychotherapy. However, these changes occurred in behaviour therapy only after improvement in phobias, whereas with group psychotherapy these changes took place irrespective of symptomatic change. There was an insignificant deterioration in family relationships at eighteen months in the individual psychotherapy patients, but at two years they were rated as improved in comparison to the start of treatment.

At the final assessment at two years conducted by a psychiatric social worker (PSW), the behaviour therapy group still showed an advantage. In symptoms, six out of sixteen were much improved and six improved. Comparable figures for group therapy were two out of sixteen and two; for individual therapy three out of ten and five. However, seven of the twelve group therapy patients without symptomatic improvement still showed improvement in social relationships. There was no evidence of symptom substitution being a particular risk of behaviour therapy. However, there were four drop-outs in the first six weeks in this group. They were replaced with well-matched new patients.

Some other interesting findings emerged from this study. Neuroticism scores on the Eysenck Personality Inventory (Eysenck and Eysenck, 1964) fell significantly in the behaviour therapy group, whereas extraversion scores rose significantly in patients receiving group psychotherapy. Agoraphobics benefited less than other types of phobia with any treatment. Other poor prognostic factors were older age at start of treatment and the presence of more neurotic symptoms.

In a cross-over study (Gelder and Marks, 1968) the seven patients who had failed to improve in group psychotherapy showed three times as much improvement in four months of desensitization as they had in the previous two years. This was a striking improvement which could not be accounted for in terms of spontaneous recovery. The fact that patients treated initially with desensitization had required an average of nine months treatment supports the finding of Lazarus (1961a) that phobias respond quicker to desensitization after patients have received group psychotherapy. It seems likely that this is due to improvement in more widespread problems resulting in the phobia becoming a more isolated symptom.

Considering the great difficulties involved in clinical research of this kind, these studies were well controlled and executed. Attention was paid to selection of patients and their assessment. Obviously no trial can claim to investigate exhaustively the efficacy of a particular treatment. There can always be uncertainty about the expertise of the therapists, the details of administration and the suitability of the selected techniques for particular patients. There is impressive evidence, however, that desensitization can bring about more rapid improvement in isolated phobias and agoraphobia of moderate severity than psychotherapy. Group psychotherapy can lead to improvement in social adjustment which may facilitate subsequent symptomatic treatment of phobias by desensitization. It remains an open question whether a comparable improvement in social adjustment could be achieved with other behaviour therapy techniques, as this was not systematically attempted in these investigations.

Because of the difficulty of exercising rigorous experimental control in the treatment of patients for whom the clinician's first concern is to administer the best treatment, a number of workers have used volunteer subjects who, although having some 'symptoms', have not sought psychiatric treatment or been referred to a psychiatrist. This is an important distinction to make, not only on account of ethical considerations, but also because there may be significant differences in the characteristics of volunteers and patients which influence the response to treatment. Both a patient and a volunteer may have a strong fear of spiders, but only a small proportion of people with a spider phobia are referred to a psychiatric clinic. It is quite probable that those who reach a psychiatrist are more distressed or restricted because of their phobia or that they have other neurotic symptoms or personality difficulties in addition which impair their social adjustment. We have already seen that these factors may have a considerable influence on the response of phobias to desensitization. Although one must be cautious in extrapolating the results of treatment of volunteers to patients, it may still be possible to investigate some aspects of therapy in this manner.

In the first attempt to explore the possibility of administering systematic desensitization on a group rather than an individual basis, Lazarus (1961a) compared group desensitization with 'more conventional forms of interpretive psychotherapy' in volunteer subjects with 'phobias'. The sample consisted of eleven agoraphobics, fifteen claustrophobics, four mixed phobias and five impotent men ('sexual phobias'). The subjects were allocated to one of three treatment regimes. Eighteen received group desensitization, nine interpretive psychotherapy and eight interpretive psychotherapy and relaxation. All patients were treated by Lazarus in groups of two to five. Thirteen out of eighteen treated with desensitization 'recovered' after an average of twenty sessions, but three had relapsed nine months later. The comparable figures for group psychotherapy with relaxation were two out of nine with one relapse, and there were no recoveries with group psychotherapy alone after an average of twenty-two sessions. In a cross-over study, ten of the fifteen subjects who had not improved in the two psychotherapy groups 'recovered' after an average of only ten sessions of group desensitization, which is half the number required by those treated with desensitization from the start.

This study is useful in demonstrating that desensitization can be conducted on a group basis and in suggesting that it may produce more rapid results in people who have already had some psychotherapy. It would be unsafe to draw any other conclusions from this study. Matching of subjects for different treatments was incomplete and the author himself carried out both assessment and treatment.

Lang and Lazovik (1963), in a well-controlled trial, studied the effects of systematic desensitization in imagination on twenty-four volunteer college students with a phobia of snakes. The students had been selected by means of a questionnaire, interview and observation of their responses to exposure to a live snake. Thirteen students formed the experimental group who had five preparatory sessions which included construction of a hierarchy, training in relaxation and imagination of scenes while under hypnosis. Half of these subjects were exposed to the snake before and after the five sessions to assess the effect of these procedures. Following the training sessions, the experimental subjects then received eleven sessions of desensitization under hypnosis. Assessment of change was made at the end of treatment and six months later. The control subjects, matched for severity of fear, received no training or desensitization but were assessed at the same time intervals as the experimental group. The experimental design thus allowed evaluation of the separate effects of repetition of an overt avoidance response to a live snake, five sessions of training in imagining scenes and relaxation, and eleven sessions of systematic desensitization itself. Only systematic desensitization had any marked effect in reducing the snake phobia, as measured by interview and reality testing, and improvement was maintained at follow-up. In addition, the amount of reduction in the fear paralleled the number of items in the hierarchy successfully desensitized.

On the basis of their findings, one would agree with the authors' conclusion that desensitization produced improvement which could not be attributed to five preparatory sessions of relaxation and hypnosis, or to suggestibility or the therapeutic relationship alone. Furthermore, they did not consider that they had altered the basic attitudes or personality of the subject whose phobia had decreased.

A later study of forty-four subjects with a fear of snakes was reported by Lang et al. (1966). Twenty-three received desensitization, ten training in relaxation and discussion of 'neutral topics' ('pseudo-psychotherapy') and eleven were untreated controls. No follow-up was undertaken, but significant reduction of the phobia occurred only in the desensitization group. One can only conclude from this experiment that desensitization is superior to some types of therapeutic relationship, relaxation, or no treatment.

Paul has carried out two excellently controlled investigations of the systematic desensitization of fear of public speaking in ninety-six college students who had high ratings in 'performance anxiety'. In the first study (Paul, 1965), subjects were assigned to one of five groups: systematic desensitization in imagination (fifteen subjects); insight oriented psychotherapy (fifteen); social attention and a placebo procedure (fifteen); untreated control group (twenty-nine); and a no-contact group. The different groups were well matched on the performance anxiety scales of a test battery. The desensitization group served as its own control by the introduction of a waiting period before the start of treatment. All therapies were carried out by five experienced psychotherapists who had been given an intensive course in behaviour therapy. Treatment consisted of five sessions of one hour spread over a six-week period. Each of the seventy-four subjects (the first four groups) was assessed before treatment by means of questionnaire, physiological measures and an independent rating of their performance in a public-speaking situation, and after treatment by physiological measures and rating in the stress situation. The desensitization group showed a significantly greater improvement than the psychotherapy and placebo-attention groups on all these measures. The improvement was maintained at a six-week follow-up on the only reassessment measure administered (questionnaires). No symptom substitution was observed. In a much more comprehensive follow-up at two years the superiority of systematic desensitization had been maintained and there was evidence of additional improvement. No evidence of symptom substitution or relapse was found (Paul, 1967).

This well-executed trial supports the findings of Lang in the previous studies discussed that desensitization is effective in reducing the fears of volunteer subjects and that this effect is not solely attributable to a therapeutic relationship or suggestion. Obviously, however, five one-hour sessions afford little test of the efficacy of insight therapy.

In another study, Paul and Shannon (1966) evaluated the effect of a modified method of desensitization. Fifty subjects, most of whom were selected from the waiting list and no-contact groups of the previous study who had shown no reduction of anxiety during the waiting period, were divided into five groups of ten. Ten subjects received group desensitization in two groups of five each. In addition they had intensive group discussion 'with re-educative goals aimed at increasing confidence, skills and awareness of effects of personal relationships'. They had nine sessions on a weekly basis and served as their own controls by the introduction of a six-week waiting period before the start of treatment. The remaining four groups of ten subjects were made up of an individual desensitization group, insight psychotherapy, attention-placebo, and a no-treatment control group. All treatment was given by the same five therapists as in the previous study. Individual treatment was restricted to five sessions over a six-week period. Similar methods of assessment were used. The results of the previous study were confirmed, with the additional finding that all the changes in the group desensitization sample 'equalled or excelled' those obtained by individual desensitization. Not only was no symptom substitution observed, but academic performance (judged by college grade points) improved significantly more in group desensitization in comparison to untreated controls. These changes had been maintained or improved at two-year follow-up assessment (Paul, 1968).

This was another well-designed and well-executed study which shows the value of desensitization in comparison to some other procedures. Group desensitization appeared more effective than individual desensitization, but further investigation would be required to confirm this, as this group had both more treatment sessions and 're-educative discussions'.

Zeisset (1968) has described a comparative trial of desensitization, relaxation and attention-placebo procedures in the treatment of patients who were anxious when interviewed. Forty-eight hospitalized patients (three 'neurotic' and forty-five 'functional psychotic') were assigned to one of four groups. The first received systematic desensitization, the second training in differential relaxation and strong suggestion that they would be able to control anxiety occurring in real-life situations, the third received attention and neutral discussion (similar to Paul's attention-placebo procedure), and the fourth was a no-treatment control group. Each treatment group had four sessions administered by one therapist. All patients were assessed before and after treatment on self-report measures, a behavioural anxiety check list completed by the ward nurses, and an observable anxiety check list completed by two independent raters during interview with the patient.

The desensitization and 'relaxation plus application' groups showed significantly greater improvement after treatment than the attention-placebo and no-treatment control groups on both observed behavioural and subjective reports of anxiety. No differences in outcome were found between the desensitization and relaxation-application groups or between the attention-placebo and no-treatment groups. The speed with which desensitization was apparently accomplished and the significantly lower frequency of anxiety signalling during desensitization are at variance with previously reported studies. However, this investigation was carried out on patients in hospital and is therefore not strictly comparable with the previous studies on volunteer subjects. Possible reasons for these findings are discussed in the next chapter.

Aversion therapy

In a comprehensive review of aversion treatment of alcoholism, Franks (1966) concluded that the majority of reports provided such inadequate information concerning procedures, controls, criteria of improvement and follow-up that claims for the efficacy of treatment are 'virtually impossible to evaluate'. Most of the studies of large series of patients which provide some adequate information have employed pharmacological rather than electrical aversive stimuli and have neglected to apply the relevant learning principles of classical conditioning to treatment. Some workers have supplemented aversion therapy with other methods so it is difficult to assess the value of aversion *per se*. The larger series report an over-all abstinence rate of about 50 per cent after various periods of follow-up. For example, Thimann (1949) treated 282 alcoholics over a period of seven years. Of 245 available for follow-up, 125 were total abstainers (including nine who had responded to further treatment after relapse). Lemere and Voegtlin (1950) included in their report 4468 patients treated over a period of thirteen years. Of these, 4096 were followed up; 44 per cent had remained totally abstinent following their first course of treatment. Eight hundred and seventy-eight relapsed cases were retreated and 39 per cent remained abstinent after this. The over-all abstinence rate was 51 per cent. In a further analysis of these results, Franks points out that 60 per cent remained abstinent for at least a year, 51 per cent two years, 38 per cent five years and 23 per cent for at least ten years after treatment. In contrast to these findings, Wallerstein (1957), comparing aversion treatment, disulfiram, group hypnosis and milieu therapy in the treatment of 178 alcoholics over a two-and-a-half year period and followed up for a year, found only 24 per cent of patients improved by aversion therapy.

Only a few studies employing electrical aversive stimuli in alcoholism have been reported. Out of forty alcoholics treated by Hsu (1965), twenty failed to complete treatment and seven of the others relapsed within six months of starting therapy. Blake (1965, 1967) published the results of a series of thirty-seven alcoholics treated with a combination of electrical aversion therapy and relaxation, and twenty-five with electrical aversion alone. All were private patients in the higher socio-economic classes. At a six-month follow-up, 52 per cent of the total sample were abstinent and 10 per cent improved. At twelve months the figures were 37 per cent and 19 per cent respectively.

There have been only a few reports of the results of aversive treatment of alcoholism with succinylcholine-induced apnoea. The number of patients treated has been small and often they have been unfavourable cases prognostically (see Madill *et al.*, 1966; Farrar *et al.*, 1968).

It is not possible to assess the value of aversion by coverant methods. Very few results of such treatment have been published. Anant (1968) has reported abstinence for a period of fourteen to twenty-one months in twenty-five out of twenty-six patients treated. Ashem and Donner (1968) obtained abstinence in a six-month follow-up in six out of fifteen patients.

Untreated alcoholism has a poor prognosis. Spontaneous remission appears to be uncommon. Of sixty-seven untreated alcoholics followed for a mean of 6·7 years, Kendall and Staton (1965) found that only one had become abstinent and fewer had returned to normal drinking than had died or committed suicide. With other forms of treatment, variable results have been attained. With 'first aid' treatment consisting of 'drying out' in hospital, the use of tranquillizers, help with personal, family and social difficulties, and encouragement to attend Alcoholics Anonymous, Vallance (1965) obtained a 5 per cent abstinence rate and 20 per cent improvement rate in sixty-eight patients followed up for two years. Davies and his colleagues (Davies *et al.*, 1956) followed up fifty alcoholics who had been admitted to hospital for two to three months and treated with disulfiram for two years. Thirty-six per cent remained abstinent for most of this period. Glatt (1961) reported a series of ninety-four alcoholics, mainly from the higher socio-economic classes, who had been in hospital and received group psychotherapy and active after-care. A two-year follow-up revealed that 66 per cent were either recovered (33 per cent) or improved. Ninety per cent of those who relapsed did so in the first six months after treatment.

Bearing in mind the quality of the available evidence, it seems that aversion therapy compares at least as favourably with other methods in the treatment of alcoholism. Further investigation may show that it may make a useful contribution to the management of this difficult disorder.

There is also very little available evidence on the results of aversion treatment in sexual deviations. Freund (1960) reported the results of apomorphine aversion in sixty-seven homosexuals. Those who were almost exclusively homosexual received a second phase of treatment aimed at establishing heterosexual interest by being shown films of nude females seven hours after they (the patients) had been given an injection of testosterone proprionate. A maximum of twenty-four aversion sessions were given, and patients who completed less than five treatment sessions were excluded from follow-up. Sixty-two were assessed three years after treatment. Of twenty patients referred from courts, only three achieved some heterosexual adaptation and this lasted only a few weeks. Of the remaining forty-seven referrals, twelve achieved some long-term adaptation although they still retained some homosexual desires, and only six claimed no overt homosexual behaviour during the follow-up period.

Apomorphine aversion treatment of nineteen transvestites reported by Morgenstern *et al.* (1965) consisted of three treatments a day for a total of thirty-nine sessions. Six out of the nineteen patients failed to complete the course. Follow-up inquiry (eight to forty-eight months) revealed that seven of the thirteen who completed treatment had stopped cross-dressing altogether and the other six had relapsed but had not returned to the same frequency of transvestite behaviour. Those who had stopped cross-dressing also showed improvement in other aspects. No symptom substitution was found.

MacCulloch and Feldman (1967) claim more encouraging results with the electric shock avoidance learning method described in the previous chapter. Thirty-six out of forty-three homosexual patients completed treatment and were followed up for at least a year. Twenty-five (56 per cent of the total sample) were considered to have improved significantly, thirteen of whom were having heterosexual intercourse unaccompanied by any homosexual practice or fantasy, seven were actively practising heterosexually but had not achieved intercourse, and five were beginning to approach active heterosexual behaviour or use strong heterosexual fantasy.

However, Bancroft and Marks (1968), reporting the results of electric aversion therapy in nineteen homosexuals and paedophiliacs, although able to obtain a high initial improvement rate (72 per cent much improved), found that only one patient had maintained this improvement at two-year follow-up and four had maintained some improvement. A better outcome was obtained with sixteen transvestites, fetishists and sadomasochists, 75 per cent of whom were much improved or improved at one-year follow-up.

Homosexuality has proved a difficult condition to treat. Although it would be premature to draw any conclusions about the efficacy of electric shock avoidance learning, these results are promising and compare favourably with other forms of treatment (e.g. Freund, 1960; Bieber et al., 1962). It seems possible that behaviour therapy methods may contribute significantly in the management of some patients with sexual deviations. The personality structure and motivation of the patient are factors which may limit the success of treatment. When the deviant sexual behaviour forms the major part of the person's sexual activity, treatment by any method is difficult.

Using aversion therapy for writer's cramp and similar disorders, Sylvester and Liversedge (1960) obtained an initial improvement (50–

100 per cent) in twenty-nine out of thirty-nine patients. Five had relapsed at follow-up which ranged from one to fifty-four months. Beech (1960) was unable to match these good results in a series of four patients who probably had more personality disturbance than those treated by Sylvester and Liversedge.

Positive conditioning

Results of behaviour treatment of nocturnal enuresis have been reviewed by Jones (1960) and Lovibond (1964). Variations in the procedure adopted, severity of the disorder, criteria of success and length of follow-up make comparison of different treatment series difficult. Jones quotes fifteen studies in which a total of 1446 enuretics (aged three to twenty-eight years) were treated with either a Mowrer or a Crosby type of apparatus, and concludes that 76 per cent (with a range of 33 –100 per cent) of the total sample recovered and 14 per cent (range 0–30 per cent) were failures. However, it is rather difficult to follow Jones's table (p. 400, 1960) summarizing these studies, as there is some ambiguity in the criteria 'cured', 'markedly improved' and 'failed', and some percentages exceed 100 per cent. Some of the figures are at variance with Lovibond's (1964) review which summarizes thirteen studies (nine of which were included in Jones's table). A total of 604 cases were treated. Initial arrest of enuresis was obtained in a median of 90 per cent (range 65 per cent to 100 per cent) of patients. The evidence concerning the relapse rate is less clear cut. The median relapse rate is quoted as 14 per cent (range 8 per cent to 52 per cent) for follow-up periods ranging from two to fifty-four months. It is apparent, however, that the longer the follow-up, the higher the relapse rate. Lovibond found a correlation of 0·7 between the reported relapse rate and the minimum period of follow-up.

Young and Turner (1965), in an investigation of the effect of stimulant drugs on conditioning procedures in enuresis, report the results on 299 children whose frequency of bedwetting was at least three nights a week. Treatment was carried out at home until fourteen consecutive dry nights had been recorded. Patients who did not achieve this criterion after four months' treatment were counted as failures. In order to assess the effects of drugs, the children were assigned to one of three treatment regimes. Detailed results of this project will be discussed in the next chapter. Here we are only concerned with the 105 children (mean age 8·1 years) who were treated with the apparatus only. The success rate was 64·8 per cent. Treatment was discontinued by 29·5 per cent and 5·7 per cent were failures because the buzzer did not wake up the children. At one year follow-up, 13·2 per cent had relapsed, but forty to sixty-three months later, of forty-one children contacted who had been dry after one year, a further 31·7 per cent had relapsed (Turner and Young, 1966).

Kahane (1955) allotted fifty-nine enuretic children to three groups. The first group of twenty-one were treated with the bell and pad. The second group of twenty-two received the same treatment after a waiting period of a few months. The third group of sixteen were examined and put on the waiting list but received no treatment. All children in the first group responded initially but thirteen out of the twenty-one relapsed within seven months. Ten out of twenty-two in the second group stopped bedwetting while on the waiting list and one relapsed. Only two children in the third group became dry and one of these relapsed.

Another controlled trial of the treatment of enuresis is that conducted by Werry and Cohrssen (1965) with seventy children. Twenty-two were allocated to treatment with the buzzer and pad, twenty-one to brief psychotherapy (nine sessions over a period of three months), and twenty-seven to a no-treatment control group. The three groups were matched for age, sex, social class, severity of enuresis and 'degree of emotional disturbance'. Treatment with the apparatus was continued until the child had been dry for at least a month or until four months of treatment were completed. At this time, improvement was observed in 80 per cent of the conditioning group as opposed to only 30 per cent in the brief psychotherapy and 30 per cent in the control groups. No symptom substitution was noticed.

The results of controlled studies suggest that a significant initial improvement can be obtained in enuresis with conditioning methods in comparison to no treatment. Unfortunately there is a significant relapse rate and we have to consider how the long-term effect of behaviour therapy compares with the spontaneous recovery rate and other forms of treatment. As yet there is insufficient evidence concerning the rate of spontaneous recovery. Lovibond (1964) states that over a twelve-month period, the percentage of spontaneous recoveries is 25 in three-year-olds and drops to 16 for eleven-year-olds. However, as Young and Turner rightly argue, the estimation of spontaneous remission rates from age incidence curves of enuresis does not take into account remissions induced by mere attendance at a clinic. As Kahane's study demonstrated, some patients recover whilst on the waiting list. Both Jones and Lovibond cite evidence that conditioning methods achieve better results than either stimulant drugs intended to reduce the depth of sleep or parasympatholytic drugs intended to inhibit micturition. Lovibond summarizes the results of psychotherapy in 195 patients in three of the most adequately reported studies. Initial arrest of enuresis was obtained in 50 per cent of children (range 25 per cent to 64 per cent). No follow-up data were reported, and at present it seems impossible to make any definitive evaluation of psychotherapy in enuresis. However, there is fairly impressive evidence that conditioning techniques are effective in obtaining initial arrest in a significant number of patients.

A variety of techniques have been employed in the treatment of stammering which influence the disorder, but there have been few published reports of the results of therapy in a series of patients. Kondas (1967b) has described the results of treatment in seventeen stammerers (aged eight to sixteen years) with shadowing techniques and relaxed breathing exercises. At the end of treatment, 70·6 per cent were rated as cured or much improved and at follow-up (minimum three years) the figure was 58·8 per cent.

Flooding or implosive therapy (IT)

It is too early to evaluate the efficacy and range of applicability of this method of behaviour therapy. As yet there have been very few published reports of treatment and they have usually involved only a handful of cases. Hogan (1966) reported encouraging results using implosive therapy as a short-term procedure with psychotic in-patients. Levis and Carrera (1967) described a controlled trial of implosive therapy in neurotic out-patients. Ten patients who received ten sessions of IT were compared with three control groups. One received 'conventional' psychotherapy for a similar number of sessions, one received an average of thirty-seven sessions of conventional psychotherapy from one of the IT therapists before he had any knowledge about IT (to control for therapist variables), and the third control group received no treatment. Ratings on the MMPI revealed significant improvement in the experimental group only. Boulougouris and Marks (1969), in a preliminary report, describe a promising response in an average of fourteen IT sessions in three out of four phobic patients (two agoraphobic and one spider-phobic); the patient who did badly was the only one with free-floating anxiety.

In a study of IT in college students with a fear of rats, fourteen out of twenty-one subjects treated were able to pick up a rat after one treatment, whereas only two out of twenty-two control subjects could do this (Hogan and Kirchner, 1967). In another study of college students with a fear of snakes (Hogan and Kirchner, 1968), ten received IT, ten 'eclectic verbal therapy' and ten 'bibliotherapy'. Seven of the ten submitted to a forty-five-minute session of IT were able to pick up a snake, in comparison with four out of ten of the eclectic verbal group and one out of ten receiving bibliotherapy. In a crossover study, ten out of the fifteen failures in the latter two treatments succeeded in picking up a snake after a forty-five-minute session of IT.

Operant conditioning

Although a great many reports of operant conditioning techniques are available, the majority of these deal with single or very few cases. Those which have included a reasonable number of patients are often experimental in nature, with the emphasis on testing the applicability of the operant conditioning model rather than actual treatment.

In their investigation of the effects of giving hospitalized chronic schizophrenic patients a programme of problem-solving tasks to perform with contingent reward of food following insulin-induced hunger, Peters and Jenkins (1954) assigned patients to three groups of twelve. One group were given injections of insulin, after which fudge was given as contingent reward for correct problem solving. Two control groups of twelve each were included. The first, controlling for the effects of insulin and personal attention, received a similar dose of insulin but were then given food which was not contingent upon completing tasks. The second control group received no treatment. Patients were assessed after the three-month experimental period and followed up for six months afterwards. Those in the experimental group improved significantly in their social behaviour, as judged by a reduction in the number of ward incidents of self-injury or violence and an increase in outings and home visits.

King *et al.* (1960) confirmed that a programme of problem-solving activities established with operant conditioning in hospitalized patients can lead to significant improvement in their clinical condition. Four groups of twelve were formed. The experimental operant group were compared with groups receiving psychotherapy, recreational therapy, and no treatment, and were found to have improved significantly more and to have maintained improvement longer than the others.

Some preliminary assessment has been made of the 'token economy' system in the ward management of hospitalized patients. Atthowe and Krasner (1968) assessed sixty patients, mostly chronic schizophrenics, during a six-month observation period and then for eleven months during the token economy regime. Thus the patients served as their own controls. Significant improvement was noted in a variety of behaviour such as taking part in group activities and going out on passes. Furthermore, twice as many patients were discharged during the eleven-month treatment period as compared with the preceding eleven months. However, half of them had to be readmitted within nine months.

Ward management along operant conditioning lines carried out by small patient groups themselves can also lead to increased sociability, shortened hospital stay and better subsequent employment record. Fairweather (1964), comparing matched groups of adult schizophrenics, eighty-four receiving 'traditional ward treatment' and 111 in small group wards, found that the latter improved significantly more when rated on these variables at follow-up. However, there was no improvement in the relapse rate. But in a second study, Fairweather *et al.* (1969) demonstrated that when the operant conditioning programme is started in hospital and then continued in a community hostel, significantly more patients maintain improvement as judged by occupational adjustment.

Schwitzgebel and Kolb (1964) evaluated the results of an operant conditioning technique in twenty adolescent delinquents compared with an untreated control group matched for age and type of first offence, nationality, religion, place of residence and duration of incarceration. The treated group received small, usually financial, rewards for good attendance, talking to a tape recorder about their personal experiences, and then for performing constructive tasks. After nine months spent in the project they left for full-time jobs, trade school or the armed forces. Follow-up three years later revealed that treatment had significantly reduced the frequency and severity of subsequent offences but not the number who had to return to prison or reformatory.

In the light of the foregoing review of the results of behaviour therapy, we can consider whether behaviour therapy 'works'. In this form the question is too broad to be answered meaningfully. It would impose homogeneity where none exists, perpetuating the mythical assumption of uniformity of patients and therapists already discussed. A more valid question to ask is what type of symptoms in which type of patients can be modified by particular methods of treatment, to what extent, and for how long. At present we can only provide partial answers with varying degrees of confidence if they are to be based on critical evidence. However, behaviour therapy is a young discipline, and attempts to evaluate its effectiveness, although rudimentary and incomplete, compare favourably with the attempts to evaluate other forms of psychological treatment. But this does not justify complacency. Further clinical and experimental studies of behaviour therapy are needed.

There is no evidence so far that behavioural methods have produced results inferior to those of other treatments in the comparative trials reviewed in this chapter. The frequency and duration of behaviour treatments are generally lower, and there is no evidence that it is a more harmful or dangerous therapy. In particular, the emergence of new symptoms, often carefully looked for because of psychoanalytical theoretical expectations, has not been found to be a special hazard. New symptoms have emerged during the course of treatment; 'social repercussions' do occur. However, they appear with no greater frequency in patients receiving behaviour therapy than other therapy or no therapy. There is difficulty in defining a 'new symptom' and assessing its relationship to the symptom being treated. This problem has been discussed recently by Crisp (1966) and Cahoon (1968), but it seems safe to conclude at present that symptom substitution has not been found to be a special risk when specific symptoms have been alleviated by behaviour therapy. This finding has important theoretical significance because, in so far as 'symptoms' are conceptualized as being the product of some underlying disorder – 'the spots of the measles' – the theory would predict that their elimination would be followed by their re-emergence or the emergence of new symptoms as long as the underlying disorders persist. Dramatic and dangerous symptom substitution has been reported in the psychiatric literature. Bookbinder (1962), for example, quotes two cases occurring after hypnotherapy and suggests that the abruptness of symptom removal may be an important variable in determining symptom substitution. However, learning principles can give some indication of the circum stances in which symptom substitution would or would not occur if certain therapeutic procedures are ignored (Cahoon, 1968).

It also seems that behaviour therapy techniques can lead to the alleviation or elimination of particular symptoms without any systematic or deliberate attempt having been made to trace their cause and development or to alter extensively the patient's personality. However, it must be borne in mind that only selected samples of patients have been submitted to behaviour therapy, usually those with relatively isolated symptoms. Results with patients with more widespread disorders have been relatively less good.

There is considerable evidence that subjects and patients with isolated phobias respond better to systematic desensitization than to other types of therapy such as individual or group psychotherapy, some forms of relaxation, suggestion and hypnosis, or no treatment. There is now some preliminary evidence that implosive (flooding) techniques and modelling (imitation) procedures may also be effective in the treatment of specific phobias. Agoraphobia of moderate severity also seems to be more responsive to desensitization than to individual or group psychotherapy. In severe agoraphobia, behaviour therapy is less efficacious but still produces slightly more favourable results than psychotherapy.

Several of the studies reviewed in this chapter cast doubt on the usefulness of Eysenck's proposal that a spontaneous remission rate of 70 per cent should be used as a baseline in assessing the results of treatment of neurosis because of the wide range of variation in outcome reported.

The evidence with regard to the efficacy of aversion therapy is less conclusive. Early attempts to treat alcoholism with pharmacological methods of aversion did not produce very impressive results. But although experience is still extremely limited, electric shock avoidance conditioning appears to be a more promising technique which can play a useful part in the treatment of transvestism, sadomasochism, fetishism and homosexuality. These are conditions usually resistant to other forms of treatment, including psychoanalysis.

Conditioning techniques appear to be the most effective method of achieving initial cessation of enuresis, but the relapse rate remains unsatisfactorily high. The few extensive clinical trials of operant techniques certainly demonstrate that they can significantly influence behaviour. Speech and social behaviour in chronic schizophrenic patients and autistic children has been improved, and this improvement has extended to behaviour outside hospital. But, heroic as some treatment programmes have been, their over-all therapeutic effect has been disappointing. Generalization of operant responses to the outside world is limited and readmission rates are little affected.

Behaviour theorists have not been unduly embarrassed by the occurrence of relapse after behaviour therapy, accounting for them in terms of learning principles. Eysenck (1963a) argues that relapse in cases of 'surplus disorders' should be infrequent because any extinction occurring as a result of random events in life works in favour of the therapist. The same learning mechanisms are invoked to explain the occurrence of new symptoms or recurrence of old symptoms as were used to explain the development of the original symptoms. However, in the case of socially disapproved behaviour treated by aversion, extinction occurring after the end of treatment will lead to the weakening of the conditioned avoidance responses which were the 'cure'. Eysenck points out that there are no empirical studies which support these hypotheses, but he thinks that clinical evidence lends some support to them. More recently Eysenck (1968a) has suggested that aversion therapy may be successful in establishing long-lasting avoidance responses in subjects in whom incubation is stronger than extinction.

In conclusion one can state that sufficient evidence has been accumulated to demonstrate that some behaviour therapy techniques have beneficial effects on certain types of psychiatric disorder. At this stage it is likely that the degree of success has been limited by the concepts and methodological requirements of controlled and experimental investigation. Theoretical considerations have led to attempts to explore particular learning models to the fullest. Those adopting the Skinnerian system, for instance, have concentrated their investigations on the clinical problems with well defined overt behavioural responses which best fit the operant paradigm. Methodological considerations demand a degree of control which encourage standardized methods of administration and the tacit ignoring of obvious individual differences. Unfortunately this must result in a somewhat narrow, strait-jacket approach. To some extent this is unavoidable. But as one tactical method, taken in conjunction with the evidence from case studies with a naturalistic approach, it can yield important information. However, if one is restricted solely to the experimental approach, the chances of discovering the full range of applicability of behaviour therapy must inevitably be diminished.

Chapter 6

Current Research I: The Specific Processes of Psychological Treatment

In the preceding chapters we have described some of the methods of behaviour therapy and their theoretical bases, and have presented some empirical evidence of their efficacy. Unfortunately, the demonstration of efficacy, even in controlled trials, neither validates the theory nor proves that the therapeutic effect is due to specific procedures involved in behaviour therapy. The therapeutic situation is always a complex one and includes such a large number of patient, therapist and therapy variables that it is inevitable that some will be disregarded in the description and analysis of treatment. Whenever a selective process is involved, such as in the choice of data to be examined in a therapeutic trial, there is a risk that our ignorance or preconceptions may prevent the discovery of significant variables. Apart from any 'specific' factors assumed to be involved in a treatment technique, there are also 'non-specific' factors such as means of referral, attendance at a clinic, diagnostic interviews, expectations concerning therapy, hospital care, suggestion, persuasion and the therapeutic relationship (see Frank, 1961). Without rigorous experimental control, therapeutic changes cannot safely be assigned to any one variable. Obviously, it is desirable to identify the crucial factors involved in successful treatment methods because this will lead to a better theoretical understanding and allow us to sharpen our therapeutic tools. In this chapter we consider some of the theoretical considerations and research investigations concerned with the role of 'specific' learning procedures in behaviour therapy. In the next chapter we review some of the evidence concerning the role of cognition and 'non-specific' factors in behaviour therapy and examine some of the other forms of psychological treatment which can have a therapeutic effect, to ascertain whether these can throw some light on the processes involved in therapeutic change.

Experimental studies of desensitization, flooding and imitation

A considerable amount of work has been focused on systematic desensitization. Broadly speaking, this has covered two aspects. The first has been concerned with an examination of the operational procedures involved, the progressive exposure to phobic stimuli, and the conditioning of an incompatible response such as relaxation. The second aspect concerns the validity of Wolpe's theoretical explanation of his method in terms of 'reciprocal inhibition'.

A great deal of research related to this problem was stimulated by Lomont (1965) who, on the basis of relevant animal studies, argued that extinction could be the underlying process involved in systematic desensitization. Obviously systematic desensitization procedures afford an opportunity for extinction to occur when conditioned phobic stimuli are presented to the patient without the subsequent reinforcement of exposure to an unconditioned aversive stimulus. Wolpe dismissed this possibility on the grounds that conditioned avoidance responses are very resistant to extinction. However, this may be due to the fact that in ordinary life the avoidance response usually prevents re-exposure to the conditioned stimuli long enough for extinction to occur. This contrasts with the treatment situation in which the patient is required to imagine the phobic stimuli for a length of time in which he is not free to make an avoidance response. Therefore the usual resistance of avoidance responses to extinction in a free situation does not exclude the possibility of extinction taking place in the treatment situation. Kimble (1961) comments that exceptions to the generally observed resistance of avoidance responses to extinction occur with embarrassing frequency.

Elucidation of this problem is not helped by ambiguity in terminology resulting from the failure to distinguish between operational procedures and theoretical constructs (see Evans and Wilson, 1968). Thus the term 'extinction' is defined as an experimental procedure, whereas 'counter-conditioning' is sometimes used as a theoretical explanation of classical extinction, and sometimes as the name of a practical procedure explicitly involving the conditioning of new responses to the CS. In view of the neurophysiological processes assumed by Wolpe to operate in 'reciprocal inhibition', this term is best reserved to describe the theoretical explanation of 'reciprocal inhibition' therapy. However, Wolpe uses the terms 'reciprocal inhibition' and 'counter-conditioning' interchangeably, so that it is not always clear in what sense they are being used. This leads to difficulty in interpreting such statements as '. . . for explaining reciprocal inhibition therapy, it is still essentially an open question as to whether the concept of reciprocal inhibition, or counter-conditioning, is more adequate than extinction' (Lomont, 1965), or 'It means also that the learning process involved is probably conditioned inhibition rather than extinction' (Rachman, 1965b).

There are usually three specific components of systematic desensitization procedures. The first involves the repeated exposure of the subject to the conditioned fear stimuli. The second involves a graduated exposure by starting with the least intense and progressing to the strongest fear stimuli. The third component is the explicit conditioning of an alternative response such as relaxation in contiguity with the CS. If the effect of systematic desensitization is contingent on repeated exposure alone (the first component), experimental extinction could account for its efficacy. If graduated exposure is found to contribute to the therapeutic effect, it would still be possible to account for its efficacy in terms of experimental extinction. However, if the third component of systematic desensitization (the evocation of an alternative response in contiguity with the fear stimulus) is found to influence therapeutic outcome, it would indicate that the effect of systematic desensitization depends on a counter-conditioning procedure whether or not extinction also plays a part.

There are several animal and human studies which are relevant to this problem. Lomont (1965) cites a number of animal experiments in which the prevention or delay of escape from a conditioned fear stimulus has led to the weakening of the previously established avoidance and fear responses. This has been achieved by confining the animal in the experimental cage, or by preventing performance of the avoidance response by curare-induced muscle paralysis. Another illustration of the effect of prolonging the exposure to the CS is provided by the ingenious experiment carried out by Delude and Carlson (1964) in which the extinction of an avoidance response in rats was hastened by a procedure which lengthened the duration of exposure to the aversive stimulus without interfering with the performance of the avoidance response.

The demonstration of anxiety reduction by flooding or implosive therapy (as described in chapter 4) is of relevance in so far as it provides evidence that procedures involving prolonged exposure to conditioned aversive stimuli without the concurrent evocation of an incompatible response can have a therapeutic effect. Lomont (1965) pointed out that confinement alone may prevent the learned avoidance response but does not necessarily lead to the extinction of conditioned fear. Duration of exposure to the fear stimulus may be a critical factor in determining whether anxiety will be increased or decreased in human subjects. Wolpin and Raines (1966) found that imagination of the most fearful items, including the criterion response of picking up the snake, for a period up to ten minutes, was successful in reducing a snake phobia. Hogan and Kirchner (1967) demonstrated the successful application of a flooding procedure in the treatment of rat phobia in which the subjects were required to imagine a series of terrifying scenes for an average of forty minutes. Rachman (1966a) failed to eliminate a phobia of spiders in three subjects who were instructed to imagine the most frightening items, but not the criterion response, for a period of two minutes. In an attempt to explain these different results, Rachman suggested that the duration, intensity and mode of presentation of the stimuli may be critical factors in producing extinction. Wolpin and Raines and Hogan and Kirchner both used more prolonged exposures than Rachman. Wilson (1967) pointed out that Wolpin and Raines instructed their subjects to imagine the successful accomplishment of the criterion response (holding a snake), whereas Rachman's subjects were required to imagine their fear responses to the most frightening items but not the criterion response. However, Hogan and Kirchner's subjects improved without imagining the actual criterion response. This has led Staub (1968) to suggest that the duration of exposure to the anxiety stimulus may be the critical factor in determining the success of flooding procedures. He considers that more prolonged exposure may lead to a state of high arousal which activates homeostatic inhibitory mechanisms. In addition, Staub suggests that more prolonged exposure may allow human subjects a better opportunity of realizing that no adverse effects result.

Obviously the question of 'reality testing' or change of expectancies is a more complex problem in implosive therapy than in desensitization. Whereas in desensitization procedures subjects imagine conditioned fear stimuli which are not dangerous in reality, implosive therapy involves imagining terrifying scenes which would be dangerous in reality. Presumably the subject learns to discriminate between imagination and reality. Stampfl assumes that all aversive stimuli experienced in imagery are secondary conditioned stimuli. The clinician is likely to be impressed by the very high levels of emotional arousal achieved in the implosive therapy methods of Stampfl, Levis, Carrera, Hogan and Kirchner and to note their resemblance to the abreactions which may occur spontaneously or during psychoanalysis, hypnotherapy or narcoanalysis. Abreaction is often followed by immediate improvement or even recovery, but unfortunately relapse occurs in a significant proportion of patients. There is some controversy concerning the theoretical basis of the therapeutic effects of abreaction. It is certainly possible that the beneficial effects of implosive therapy depend upon the extinction of fear responses as a result of the identification and imagination of the specific aversive stimuli which evoked them. But the alternative explanation, that abreaction or catharsis may have a non-specific effect in relieving anxiety and other neurotic symptoms which is dependent upon the level of emotional arousal and its expression, rather than by the actual content of the fantasies, has to be considered. Empirical evidence obtained by a comparison of abreaction with and without the use of specific phobic stimuli might throw some light on this issue. Further studies will also be required to control for the strong placebo effect which a dramatic and frightening treatment would be expected to have.

The animal and human studies discussed so far indicate that delaying the escape from a conditioned aversive stimulus can lead to the extinction of avoidance and fear responses without the addition of an overt counterconditioning procedure. Flooding and implosive techniques which involve the prolonged exposure of the subject to conditioned fear stimuli can facilitate extinction of anxiety. However, systematic desensitization and counterconditioning procedures provide for the elicitation and strengthening of an alternative response as well as exposure to the conditioned fear stimulus. Does the addition of a counterconditioning technique lead to a greater reduction in anxiety than could be accounted for on the basis of extinction alone?

A few attempts have been made to carry out controlled comparisons of counterconditioning and extinction procedures. In one study, Gale *et al.* (1966) submitted eighteen rats to a classical conditioning procedure in which a tone was paired with a strong shock. Defecation was used as an objective measure of conditioned fear. Three matched groups were formed on the basis of the weight of faeces excreted. Group 1 received an extinction procedure in which a succession of tones gradually approximating the original CS were presented. Group 2 received the same procedure with the addition of food as a stimulus for a response incompatible with anxiety. Group 3 were a control for the passage of time alone. Group 2 showed a significantly faster reduction of conditioned fear (as measured by defecation) than Group 1, but the extinction procedure also led to a significant reduction of fear in comparison with the control group. The results of this study indicate that under these experimental conditions, a counterconditioning procedure is superior to an extinction procedure alone. However, no difference was found in the rate of reconditioning the original fear response. A possible explanation of this may have been that the counterconditioning group had stopped responding earlier than the extinction group in the deconditioning procedures, and therefore received many 'over-extinction' trials.

Gambrill (1967) carried out an experiment to compare the efficacy of a counterconditioning procedure and an extinction procedure in eliminating an avoidance response. Forty-three rats were trained to turn a wheel in order to avoid the next scheduled shock. Following this, the rats were matched according to their rate of avoidance responding and randomly allocated to one of five groups. Group 1 were trained to raise a lever to obtain food and then submitted to a counterconditioning procedure in which the lever response was still reinforced with food while no shocks were administered for failure to turn the wheel. Group 2 were treated in the same way except that during counterconditioning trials the lever response was not reinforced. Group 3 were initially treated in the same way but then had no opportunity of performing the lever response (the lever was absent). The rats in Group 4 were exposed to the lever initially but not trained to raise the lever for reinforcement; during extinction trials the lever was present. Group 5 received no special training and were submitted to a straightforward classical extinction procedure.

Only the counterconditioning procedure (Group 1), in which an alternative response was available and received reinforcement, proved more effective than the classical extinction procedure (Group 5) in reducing the rate of avoidance responding. This effect was evident only in the first session and, when the competing response was eliminated by removal of the lever after the third trial, only the animals in Group 1 showed a significant increase in avoidance responses. Furthermore, all procedures succeeded in eliminating avoidance behaviour after ten extinction trials. The extent of the delay was related to the degree to which a procedure introduced a competing response. Hence this study lends further support to Gale's findings that a counterconditioning procedure effects a significantly faster reduction in avoidance response rate than an extinction procedure. Both studies indicate that an extinction procedure alone can cause some reduction in avoidance behaviour, but Gambrill's experiment suggests that a counterconditioning procedure, like punishment combined with an extinction procedure, produces an immediate suppression in the rate of responding, but when the new response is prevented an increase in the avoidance response occurs.

Gambrill did not employ a gradual presentation of the stimuli associated with the avoidance response. Lomont points out that this 'progressive principle' is a prominent feature of 'reciprocal inhibition' procedures which has not received adequate investigation. Most of the animal studies in this area have been concerned with the extinction of the most fearful stimulus rather than the entire anxiety hierarchy. In an experiment not cited by Lomont, Kimble and Kendall (1953) demonstrated that rats submitted to extinction trials in which the cs (light) was repeatedly presented in its original intensity showed a slower diminution in avoidance responses than rats exposed to the cs light at a gradually increasing intensity.

An experiment conducted by Agras (1965) supports Lomont's thesis that an extinction process may occur in 'reciprocal inhibition' procedures. During the systematic desensitization of six phobics a considerable degree of 'spontaneous recurrence' of anxiety was observed (measured by skin resistance) in response to the presentation of previously successfully completed items. Spontaneous recovery, Lomont comments, is a familiar phenomenon in extinction, whereas it is difficult to account for in counterconditioning when elimination of the old response is due to its replacement by a new one.

On the basis of the human and animal studies reviewed so far, we would agree with Lomont's earlier view (1965) that the extent to which the efficacy of Wolpe's systematic desensitization procedure depends on counterconditioning or extinction remains uncertain. More recent studies with human subjects, however, have tended to emphasize the contribution of counterconditioning.

Lomont and Edwards (1967) carried out an experiment to determine whether the efficacy of systematic desensitization depended upon the contiguity of muscular relaxation and imagination of the anxiety situation, and whether the therapeutic effect was more satisfactorily explained in terms of counterconditioning or extinction. The study employed a complex design and was tightly controlled. Twenty-two female college students with a phobia of snakes were divided into two treatment groups. One group received systematic desensitization which differed from the usual procedures in that while imagining each anxiety item the subjects were required to sustain a mild degree of muscular tension which was standardized mechanically. The end of imagining the scene or the signalling of anxiety, whichever came first, was followed by twenty seconds of relaxation. The other group received a similar procedure except that relaxation was omitted (extinction procedures). The results of the study revealed that on three out of five measures of anxiety, systematic desensitization produced significantly or nearly significantly greater reduction than did the extinction procedure which appeared totally ineffective.

Davison (1968c) investigated the treatment of college students with a fear of snakes. Twenty-eight subjects were matched in terms of the intensity of their avoidance of snakes and allocated to one of four regimes. Eight students received systematic desensitization in the usual manner. Eight received 'pseudo-desensitization' which was identical to the first except that essentially neutral and irrelevant childhood scenes were used as the imaginal scenes paired with relaxation. The third group of eight subjects were presented with the same items of the snake hierarchy as the systematic desensitization group, but without relaxation. The fourth group, consisting of only four students, were given no treatment. Subjects in the second and third groups were 'yoked' to their matched partners in the systematic desensitization group to ensure that all received the same duration and number of sessions and stimulus exposures. All subjects were assessed before and after the experiment on a snake-avoidance test (similar to that used by Lang and Lazovik, 1963) and on a ten-point self-rating anxiety scale. The same therapist carried out all the treatments, a maximum of nine sessions were given, and assessments were carried out by an experimenter who did not participate in the treatment.

The results of this experiment revealed that only subjects submitted to systematic desensitization showed a significant reduction in avoidance behaviour and rating of anxiety. Five out of eight had completed the anxiety hierarchy within the nine sessions, and four were able to perform the top item of holding the snake. There was slight but nonsignificant improvement in the pseudo-desensitization group, and only one of the subjects was able to hold a snake at the end of treatment. None of the students in the exposure or no-treatment groups were able to hold a snake or showed improvement. It was noticed that subjects in the exposure group signalled anxiety much more often during treatment sessions than subjects in the desensitization group. A correlation of 0·81 was obtained between anxiety reduction and approach behaviour, indicating that subjects who experience the greatest amount of anxiety reduction also displayed the greatest increment in approach behaviour.

This well-controlled study demonstrated that neither graded exposure alone nor relaxation alone was effective in reducing fear and avoidance behaviour, but the combination of the two was effective. The author concluded that his findings supported 'the hypothesis that behavioural changes produced by systematic desensitization reflect a counterconditioning process', in that it is the association of anxiety-inhibiting relaxation responses with the phobic stimuli which yields significant changes. This study also confirms the efficacy of systematic desensitization in the treatment of isolated fears in volunteers and affords some indirect evidence that this cannot be accounted for on the basis of the subject's expectancy of improvement or interaction with a therapist alone.

Rachman (1965b) has investigated the same problem using a similar experimental design. Twelve volunteer subjects with a fear of spiders were allocated to one of four treatment groups: systematic desensitization, graded presentation of aversive stimuli without relaxation, relaxation alone, and no-treatment controls. Again, a significant reduction of fear was obtained only in the systematic desensitization group, and this was maintained at three-month follow-up. Rachman's conclusions, more tentatively expressed in view of the small number of subjects, are virtually the same as those of Davison. But he points out that these results do not imply that extinction is never responsible for the reduction of fear, but that 'in the present context, however, inhibition is a more effective process'.

Another similar investigation conducted by Kondas (1967a), compared systematic desensitization, gradual exposure, and relaxation procedures in the treatment of twenty-three schoolchildren and thirteen psychology students who appeared to experience excessive fear of school or college examinations. Treatment was carried out in groups and assessment was rated by means of a fear schedule and palmar skin sweating under school examination conditions. In general his results corroborate those of Davison and Rachman with the exception that a significant improvement was also recorded on the fear questionnaire in children who received relaxation alone. Unfortunately, this study was not well controlled. There was no attempt to match the different treatment groups for intensity of anxiety, the number of treatment sessions was not held constant, children in the 'relaxation only' group were in fact requested to practise relaxation in the classroom also, and the validity of the assessment procedures is uncertain. It is possible, therefore, that the improvement noted on the fear schedule in the group receiving relaxation may be due to the contamination in the experimental design. However, Zeisset (1968), in the study quoted in the previous chapter, also found that a relaxation procedure effectively reduced anxiety (interview anxiety in hospitalized psychiatric patients). In view of the fact that Zeisset did not attempt to countercondition a new response in his 'relaxation plus application' group, it is difficult to explain its efficacy. It seems highly unlikely that suggestion would play a significant part since the attention-placebo group did not improve. Davison (1969) suggested that the differential relaxation training, if successful, enabled subjects to feel that they were reducing their own anxieties and to experience self-control. Awareness of this ability could lead to the subject practising relaxation between treatment sessions when in the presence of the phobic or related anxiety stimuli and so desensitizing himself.

Cooke (1968) compared the efficacy of systematic desensitization, graded presentation of hierarchy items without relaxation, and relaxation alone in reducing fear of rats. Fifty volunteer college students were divided into five groups of ten. The first had one session of training in relaxation and hierarchy construction followed by five sessions of systematic desensitization. The second group had five sessions of graded presentation without relaxation after the preliminary session of training in relaxation and hierarchy construction. The third group had a preliminary session of training in relaxation and hierarchy construction followed by five sessions of relaxation. The fourth group had only one session of hierarchy construction, the fifth had no treatment. The fear of rats was rated by questionnaire (FSS) and an avoidance test assessed by three independent judges. The results showed that both systematic desensitization and graded presentation alone produced significant improvement. As in Lang and Lazovik's study (1963), subjects who had completed the hierarchy showed the most improvement. Cooke comments that an extinction process would account better than counterconditioning for this therapeutic result. Certainly one would expect the systematic desensitization procedure to be superior if counterconditioning plays a significant role in treatment. However, it is quite possible that counterconditioning did occur during the graded presentation sessions because the subjects had been trained in relaxation in the preliminary session and may therefore have covertly relaxed themselves during the presentation of the items or felt calm in the presence of the experimenter. In any event, they were instructed to signal if they felt anxious and items were presented until no anxiety was evoked. Counterconditioning could occur during this procedure.

Specific Processes

In a rather different context, Folkins *et al.* (1968) found that imagination of items without relaxation (cognitive rehearsal) was superior to an approximate analogue of systematic desensitization or relaxation in reducing the amount of anxiety evoked by a film depicting a fatal accident. This at least suggests that procedures other than systematic desensitization can reduce emotional responses. Obviously this investigation did not provide an adequate test of systematic desensitization.

Evidence concerning the effective processes involved in systematic desensitization in a rather different setting is provided by Moore (1965), who set out to compare the effects of systematic desensitization, relaxation and suggestion and relaxation alone in twelve consecutive asthmatic patients referred to a general hospital chest clinic. In the systematic desensitization procedure, three hierarchies were used. One consisted of items concerned with an actual asthmatic attack, one was made up of situations which incorporated relevant allergic or infective factors, and the final one was composed of psychologically stressful situations derived from 'the psychodynamic formulation'. In the relaxation and suggestion procedure, the patients were trained in deep relaxation and given suggestions that they would improve in various specified ways. All patients were instructed to practise relaxation at home. Moore employed a balanced incomplete block design, using patients as their own controls. There were six blocks covering every combination and sequence of treatments. Each of the blocks was given to one adult and one child, randomly allocated. Each patient received two of the three treatment procedures in two courses of weekly sessions of eight weeks' duration, with a one-week rest period between them. The effects of treatment were assessed by a combination of the patients' subjective report of frequency of asthmatic attacks and objective measurement of ventilation. Subjective improvement was reported initially in all the treatment groups, but whereas this increased gradually in the desensitization group, it declined with the other groups. Objective improvement in ventilation also occurred with all the treatment procedures, but significantly more with desensitization. As each patient received two treatments, the experiment does not lend itself to assessment of follow-up results. However, no patient who received desensitization relapsed during a six-month period following treatment.

This is an important study because patients rather than non-patient volunteer subjects were used, and it is the first controlled investigation of the efficacy of systematic desensitization in bronchial asthma. Unfortunately, the design of the experiment imposes limitations on the conclusions which can be drawn. It does not allow an accurate assessment of the possible effect of the first treatment on the second one. Furthermore, although the study demonstrates the superiority of systematic desensitization over relaxation alone or relaxation plus suggestion, it does not isolate the effect of graded exposure from that of relaxation. In view of this the author is not really justified in her conclusion that 'reciprocal inhibition is found to be the crucial factor in desensitization'.

Marks *et al.* (1968) compared the effects of systematic desensitization with those of suggestion during relaxation induced by hypnosis in phobic patients. Twenty-eight out-patients were allocated randomly to the two treatment procedures. The group receiving systematic desensitization were instructed to practise in real life the items they could imagine without anxiety. The other group received forceful general suggestions of improvement while under hypnosis. They were not asked to imagine specific phobic situations or to practise graduated tasks in real life. Both groups received twelve treatment sessions at weekly intervals. After a six-week delay, patients who had not shown improvement received a twelve-week course of the alternative treatment. At the end of the crossover treatment, twenty-three patients had received desensitization and eighteen hypnosis.

Progress in treatment was rated by the patient, therapist and an independent assessor before, during and after treatment, and at one year on scales of symptom severity and social adjustment. A psychiatric social worker interviewed patients at the beginning and end of treatment and also at one year follow-up. Some symptom and personality inventories and three measures of suggestibility were completed before the start of treatment.

The results showed that both treatments produced significant improvement in the treated phobias. Although all raters agreed that desensitization produced more improvement than hypnosis, only one set of ratings showed a significant difference. Statistical analysis of twenty-nine variables failed to identify any of prognostic value. An item analysis of the previously established prognostic questionnaire (Gelder *et al.*, 1967), also failed to reveal any useful prognostic items in this study. However, there was a significant correlation between introversion and improvement with hypnosis.

Marks *et al.* (1968) appear to be somewhat puzzled by their failure to demonstrate a significant difference between systematic desensitization and hypnotic suggestion in the treatment of phobic patients. In their discussion of the reasons for this, they suggest, on the basis of previous therapeutic trials, that ratings at twenty-four weeks might have shown a significant difference. In addition they point out that suggestions may operate in part by reducing anticipating anxiety so that the patient can enter phobic situations and undergo practical retraining. It is also possible that some patients actually imagined phobic scenes while under hypnotic relaxation so that desensitization in imagination could have taken place. Obviously suggestion during relaxation has some therapeutic effect but the consistent results in this and other studies in favour of systematic desensitization indicate that suggestion, by whatever mechanisms, is not responsible for all its effect.

Although the experimental studies of systematic desensitization in human subjects have produced somewhat conflicting results, the evidence tends to suggest that the combination of relaxation and gradual presentation of phobic stimuli produces the best result. When this is the case, systematic desensitization cannot be accounted for on the basis of classical extinction alone, but a counterconditioning process must be involved. Obviously, these conclusions are only applicable to systematic desensitization procedures, and not to flooding or implosive techniques.

At first sight it might appear that systematic desensitization and flooding are completely opposite procedures which could not be derived from the same learning principles. Certainly one procedure aims to inhibit or suppress any anxiety from being experienced by the patient, while the other attempts to elicit and maintain a maximal level of anxiety. But this is because the rationale of the two procedures is different. One is based on counterconditioning, the other on extinction by non-reinforced practice. It is no abuse of logic to postulate the existence of more than one process by which learned responses can be modified. The clinician would like to know whether counterconditioning or extinction procedures are the more effective and whether the method of choice is dependent on the type of patient and disorder to be treated. Acquisition and extinction are affected differently by variables such as drugs and massed as opposed to distributed practice, and these would be manipulated by the therapist according to the principle of treatment adopted.

Ramsay *et al.* (1966) compared the effects of massed and distributed trials in the systematic desensitization of various animal phobias in twenty volunteer psychology students. Massed treatment consisted of two forty-minute sessions (one per day), spaced treatment four twenty-minute sessions (one per day). All subjects were submitted to both procedures with half receiving one the first week and the other the second week. Both procedures produced a significant reduction of fear, but spaced practice was significantly superior (5 per cent level for one tail test). This is consistent with other experimental evidence of the beneficial influence of spaced practice on learning and appears consistent with the notion that desensitization involves a counterconditioning process.

Attempts have also been made to investigate several other aspects of systematic desensitization. It is generally assumed by behaviour therapists that the anxiety response to every item should be reduced to zero during treatment. According to Wolpe's principle of reciprocal inhibition, however, either complete or partial suppression of anxiety is sufficient. Rachman and Hodgson (1967) attempted to investigate the degree of anxiety reduction which has to be achieved before proceeding to the next item in the hierarchy. Ten volunteer subjects with a phobia of spiders were divided into two groups, matched for the initial intensity of fear. A subjective rating of fear ('fear thermometer') was obtained for each item initially and after every third presentation. In the first group, anxiety was reduced to zero on every item, whereas in the second group only a 50 per cent reduction in anxiety was obtained. Results, assessed by an objective avoidance test and subjective anxiety ratings, revealed that complete suppression of anxiety was not significantly superior and the partial suppression treatment took less time.

Theoretical as well as practical issues are raised by the apparent efficacy of partial suppression of anxiety. Further experimental evidence is required to confirm this (see Beech, 1969). If a new response of relaxation can be established in the presence of some anxiety, relaxation and anxiety are not incompatible responses. If this is the case, it is difficult to know why relaxation does not come to evoke anxiety as a result of systematic desensitization therapy. Some authors have examined critically the assumption that muscular relaxation inhibits anxiety. Wolpe (1958) accepted Jacobson's reasoning (1938, 1964) that deep muscular relaxation inhibits anxiety because the reduction in feedback of proprioceptive impulses from relaxed muscles is incompatible with the experience of anxiety. But Davison (1966) has drawn attention to various animal studies in which fear responses were established despite complete drug-induced muscle paralysis. Subjective anxiety is reported by human subjects paralysed with scoline and this has been employed as an aversive stimulus. This evidence is inconsistent with the views of Jacobson and Wolpe. Davison suggests that there may be a difference between self-induced and drug-induced muscular relaxation and tentatively puts forward two hypotheses to account for the reduction in anxiety achieved by training in muscular relaxation. The first derives from the observation that a variety of responses incompatible with anxiety have been used in 'reciprocal inhibition' procedures, including feeding, sexual, assertive and emotive imagery as well as muscular relaxation. These incompatible responses may all have in common the ability to generate positive affective states. Self-induced muscular relaxation may well be able to induce a positive affect which drug-induced paralysis could not. The second hypothesis suggests that inhibitory efferent motor impulses which mediate self-induced muscle relaxation (but not curare paralysis) may be responsible for the inhibition of anxiety.

Obviously the affective state of the subject might be more relevant than his muscle tone. The procedures employed to obtain muscle relaxation include an element of suggestion, and some procedures specifically aim at producing an hypnotic state. Rachman (1968) makes the same points as Davison and points out that although relaxation appears to be a necessary component of desensitization, there is no convincing evidence that muscular relaxation is essential. He points out that therapeutic effects have been obtained when patients are physically active in practical retraining or after only very brief training in relaxation. Furthermore, there is some evidence that during relaxation induced by Wolpian methods, the subjects' reports of calmness are not always accompanied by decreased electromyographic activity (Gelder, 1968). There is a large body of evidence that verbal suggestion designed to evoke particular emotional states can also lead to the appropriate changes in physiological functions.

Tranquillizer and sedative drugs have also been employed to induce relaxation. In an attempt to investigate the efficacy of methohexitone desensitization, Yorkston *et al.* (1968) studied twelve hospitalized patients with severe agoraphobia. In order to isolate the effect of methohexitone, four procedures were used. In the first procedure, desensitization was carried out with methohexitone relaxation (verbal suggestions of relaxation were avoided). The second procedure consisted of desensitization with verbal relaxation and injection of saline, the third was desensitization without any injection, while the fourth consisted of methohexitone injections without desensitization. A balanced incomplete block design was employed with each patient receiving two of the four procedures (one hour daily for five days). The patients were assessed by an independent judge before and after each procedure by means of questionnaires, rating scales and an avoidance test. The results showed that no groups improved significantly. The authors conclude that this does not suggest that methohexitone desensitization is necessarily the treatment of choice for severely agoraphobic in-patients. One must agree with their conclusion but it is difficult to understand why this was 'contrary to expectations'. On the clinical evidence available on the treatment of severe agoraphobic in-patients (e.g. Gelder and Marks, 1966), it seems optimistic to expect that five one-hour sessions of desensitization would be sufficient to produce significant improvement. In the design of a therapeutic trial an attempt should be made to include a procedure which is capable of having a positive effect if false negative conclusions are to be avoided (Laurence, 1962). However, in a useful introduction to their paper, Yorkston *et al.* (1968) comment that 'systematic desensitization' is used in two senses. The first has a wider connotation, including the establishment of rapport, discussion of aetiology, explanation of treatment, encouragement and interest in the patient's pattern of recovery as well as systematic desensitization and practical retraining. The second meaning of 'systematic desensitization' has the narrower connotation of systematic desensitization in imagination alone. In this study it appears that an attempt was made to study the effect of systematic desensitization in the narrower sense. The relative contributions of systematic desensitization in imagination and practical retraining in the treatment of phobias remain uncertain. Some of the experimental evidence is discussed later in this chapter and the problems involved in the assessment of the 'non-specific' factors in systematic desensitization (in its wider sense) are discussed in the next chapter.

Although muscular relaxation may not be essential in systematic desensitization and a state of calm or relaxation can be induced by suggestion, hypnosis or drugs, it would seem premature to abandon this procedure yet. Most of the evidence of the efficacy of systematic desensitization in psychiatric patients has been with muscular relaxation. It is quite possible that muscular relaxation is the most effective method of inducing a state of calm in neurotic subjects. Further investigation will determine whether this is the method of choice.

Lader and Wing (1966) have put forward a different theoretical interpretation of the process of desensitization in psychiatric patients which is relevant to the problem of the importance of muscular relaxation, and indeed the whole principle of counterconditioning. In a series of experiments attempting to discover reliable indices of anxiety which would discriminate between normal and anxious subjects, and which would be sensitive to sedative drugs, they found that spontaneous fluctuation of skin resistance at rest (PGR) and the rate of decrement of PGR to repeated identical auditory stimuli (habituation) met these criteria. The rate of habituation in patients suffering from morbid anxiety was inversely related to the level of arousal as reflected by the amount of spontaneous fluctuation of the PGR. When arousal is high, habituation is slow, particularly at the outset, whereas when it is low habituation proceeds more rapidly. If the subject is over-aroused each successive presentation of the stimulus leads to increasing levels of activity and no habituation takes place. They suggest that the speed of habituation of a particular subject at a given time depends on two variables, an innate habituation property and the level of arousal at the time. With a 'fast habituator' a repetitive stimulus raises activity initially but falls as habituation takes place. With a 'slow habituator', repetitive stimulus presentation leads to increasing activity and increasingly slow habituation. Similarly the level of arousal influences habituation. At low levels, habituation proceeds rapidly, whereas at high levels, not only does habituation fail to occur but the GSR increases as the stimulus presentation is repeated. Lader and Mathews (1968) suggest that there is a critical level of arousal above which habituation will not occur and anxiety will increase to panic if the patient is subjected to repeated exposure to his phobic stimulus.

On the basis of these findings and theoretical considerations, Lader and Wing postulated that therapeutic 'systematic desensitization' was due to habituation to phobic stimuli occurring at a low level of arousal induced by relaxation. Consistent with this interpretation is the finding by Lader (1967) that patients with monosymptomatic phobias resemble normal controls in showing less spontaneous fluctuation in GSR and faster habituation than patients with anxiety states, social phobias or agoraphobia. Furthermore, fast habituators respond better to desensitization (Lader *et al.*, 1967) which is in keeping with the clinical finding that simple phobias respond best to this type of treatment. The observed correlation between isolated phobias, absence of generalized anxiety and panic attacks, low levels of arousal, rapid habituation, and response to treatment by systematic desensitization certainly suggests that habituation could be the process responsible for therapeutic change.

In addition, there is some evidence that reducing high levels of anxiety can facilitate subsequent systematic desensitization. Tranquillizing and sedative drugs or carbon dioxide inhalations have been employed in patients with free floating anxiety. Friedman and Silverstone (1967) reported the successful use of methohexitone, and Yeung (1968) has recommended the use of diazepam. There is also some evidence that prefrontal leucotomy, which reduces generalized anxiety (Levinson and Meyer, 1965; Marks *et al.*, 1966), has been followed by the successful desensitization of obsessional symptoms which had not responded previously to this treatment (Walton and Mather, 1963). Marks *et al.* (1966) refer to one phobic patient who improved with desensitization following leucotomy.

Specific Processes

Lader and Mathews (1968), argue, on the basis of some theoretical considerations and selected experimental evidence, that the model of habituation at low arousal accounts better for the effects of systematic desensitization than Wolpe's theory of reciprocal inhibition. However, their points do not appear compelling and they themselves admit that further experimental investigation is required. Marks *et al.* (1968) suggest that a number of variables may contribute to the therapeutic outcome of systematic desensitization and that in patients with low levels of anxiety, habituation and counterconditioning may be more important than suggestion, whereas at higher levels of arousal, suggestion may play a more important role.

Obviously the combination of relaxation and repetitive presentation of stimuli in systematic desensitization procedures provide an opportunity for habituation to take place. At first sight there appears to be a considerable difference between the description of systematic desensitization in terms of habituation at low levels of arousal as opposed to counterconditioning and extinction as previously discussed. Lader and Wing emphasize 'low arousal', whereas 'counterconditioning' emphasizes more the procedures whereby 'low arousal' is presumably achieved. Lader and Wing refer to phobic response decrement as 'habituation' in preference to 'extinction'. It is difficult to know whether the difference in the two descriptions is at a semantic, theoretical, neurological or psychological level. There is some confusion in terminology, but the term 'habituation' has usually been restricted to the decrement of unconditioned responses (such as the orientation and startle reflexes) following the repeated presentation of a stimulus (Galambos and Morgan, 1960; Thompson and Spencer, 1966), and has not included the decrement of conditioned responses evoked by conditioned stimuli. Sokolov (1963) described the different time course of the orientation and conditioned responses during conditioning procedures and the more temporary effect of habituation. At the level of behavioural analysis, Thompson and Spencer consider that habituation and extinction share nine parametric characteristics and may therefore be identical processes, with the exception that extinction implies prior conditioning. It seems likely that the two procedures must involve similar if not identical neurophysiological processes, but as these have not yet been fully delineated (see, for

174

instance, Kimble, 1961; Glaser, 1966; Stein, 1966), there may be some advantage in retaining the separate operational definitions of habituation and experimental extinction. We are not qualified to review critically the physiological theories concerning habituation and extinction. However, that it may be wise to keep the terms separate on clinical grounds is illustrated by Napalkov's (1963) experiment in which dogs habituated to the repeated presentation of an unconditioned aversive stimulus, but not to the repeated presentation of a conditioned aversive stimulus alone, which resulted in a sustained rise in blood pressure persisting for over sixteen months despite 900 extinction trials. If one argues that the dogs were too highly aroused to 'habituate' to the cs, it is difficult to see why they should have habituated to the ucs. Furthermore, the evidence showing that non-psychiatric subjects, not generally characterized by high arousal levels, tend to respond less well to procedures involving a gradual presentation of 'phobic' stimuli without relaxation argues against the habituation hypothesis. Perhaps the apparent efficacy of flooding, which presumably evokes very high levels of arousal, also suggests that mechanisms other than habituation at low levels of arousal can reduce or eliminate anxiety responses.

Although it would be premature to draw definitive theoretical conclusions, clinical considerations suggest that we still adopt a counterconditioning model. As already discussed, the bulk of the clinical and experimental evidence favours counterconditioning procedures rather than experimental extinction alone as being the most effective ingredient of systematic desensitization.

Apart from these explanations, another account of the process of desensitization has been put forward by Valins and Ray (1967), who derived their theoretical model from cognitive theories of emotion (Schachter, 1964). Subjects undergoing systematic desensitization are motivated to re-evaluate their phobic attitudes and behaviour because they realize that a previously arousing stimulus has no physiological effect. Two groups of university students matched in respect of fear of snakes and electric shock were assigned to a control and an experimental group. The experimental group were shown slides of the word 'shock' and concurrent mild electric shock to their fingers and ten slides of snakes. They heard what they thought were their heart rate reactions (faked) to these slides. Heart rate was not affected by the snake slides but increased when shock was administered. Control subjects were exposed to the same slides and faked heart rates but were informed that the latter was just extraneous noise. Subsequent snake-avoidance test showed a significant improvement in snake-approach behaviour by the experimental group. In a second experiment they selected students who exhibited more than average fear of snakes. Instead of slides, a live snake in a glass cage was used. Otherwise the procedure employed was similar. Significant improvement in approach behaviour was again obtained in the experimental group. This is an interesting study. However, one would have to exclude the possibility that hearing the monotonous beat of one's own heart beat could induce relaxation and therefore counterconditioning. Secondly, one cannot conclude on the basis of the available evidence that pronounced changes in the experimental subjects' heart rate could not be detected. Finally, although there is sufficient evidence to indicate the importance of cognitive processes for the experience of emotions, it is still necessary to demonstrate that similar results could be obtained with psychiatric patients suffering from severe phobias if it is to be of clinical value.

Further experimental investigations have been carried out to determine the time course of reduction in anxiety and autonomic responses following desensitization. Lazarus and Rachman (1960) drew attention to a time lag in the effects of desensitization. Some patients only noticed a reduction of their anxiety response to specific phobic stimuli some time after these had been desensitized in imagination. Lang and Lazovik (1963) found that subjective reports of improvement lagged behind objective change in avoidance behaviour. Avoidance-test scores discriminated treated from control subjects immediately after treatment, but this was not reflected in subjective ratings until the follow-up assessment. It seems possible that a similar discrepancy between objective and subjective improvement may have occurred in the patients studied by Lazarus and Rachman.

Clearly, the degree of generalization to real life situations as well as the speed of anxiety reduction is crucial to therapeutic success in psychiatric patients (see Hain *et al.*, 1966; Meyer and Crisp, 1966). Davison (1968c) points out that on theoretical grounds a complete transfer from imagined scenes to real life situations would not be expected because anxiety hierarchies are unlikely to include all the elements involved in a patient's phobia. Two attempts have been made to throw some light on these problems.

Rachman (1966b) has studied the speed of generalization from desensitization in imagination to real life stimuli. The main aims were 'to search for time-lags and to pin down the time at which generalization occurs'. Also of therapeutic importance is the timing and incidence of relapse after treatment. 'Spontaneous recurrence' of anxiety to items already successfully desensitized was reported by Agras (1965). Rachman studied three volunteer spider phobic subjects who were exposed to an anxiety provoking stimulus involving spiders and required to rate their degree of fear. They were then desensitized to the identical stimulus used in the initial avoidance test and reassessed on the same measures (avoidance test and fear rating) immediately after treatment and again twenty-four hours, three days or a week later. Judged by fear ratings, immediate transfer from imagined to real life stimuli occurred to some extent in 82 per cent of observations. The transfer was never complete and in a small proportion of cases an increase in fear was rated after desensitization of intense anxiety items. Immediate reductions in anxiety were not always stable and some degree of relapse occurred in about 40 per cent of observations. In some cases, however, further improvement took place during the follow-up period. The study did not throw light on the factors which influence the stability of anxiety reduction.

The exploratory nature of this investigation precludes any firm conclusions. Further investigations with psychiatric patients are required. Desensitization followed by immediate assessment with identical stimuli in a limited and rather artificial laboratory situation may have given rise to a spuriously high amount of generalization. Agras (1967) argues that patients with phobic symptoms do not usually expose themselves to the feared situation immediately after each desensitization session and would not therefore profit from the effects of immediate transfer. On a practical level, Rachman's findings support those of Agras (1965) in that some subjects exhibited a partial recurrence of anxiety responses to items already successfully desensitized in previous sessions. Agras suggests that this may be one explanation for clinical relapse following desensitization and indicates that all items of the hierarchy should be completely desensitized. Reinforcement of an anxiety response to a partially desensitized item could lead to generalization and total relapse. The therapist should check at the start of each treatment session that desensitization to all the items already treated has been maintained. Relevant in this connexion are Wolpe's findings (1963) which show that the number of times a scene has to be presented before anxiety is eliminated is not the same for all items. When fear increases in proportion to proximity to the phobic stimulus (e.g. animals), the number of desensitization trials increases with proximity. On the other hand, in phobias in which anxiety increases with distance from a safe place (e.g. agoraphobia) the number of presentations required is high initially, but gradually diminishes. The same phenomenon was observed in Rachman's study (1966b).

Agras (1967) investigated the problem of transfer using five agoraphobic patients. Progress in desensitization was expressed as the percentage change in the cumulative number of scenes imagined without anxiety being signalled. Generalization of anxiety reduction in two different test situations was explored. In the first the patient imagined five items from the anxiety hierarchy before the start of a desensitization session and the degree of anxiety evoked was measured by change in log conductance of GSR (corrected for baseline variation). The second situation was the patient's performance in the actual feared situation obtained from a detailed self-report of distance travelled. Between fifteen and seventy sessions were required to reach the criterion of improvement. Four of the patients were improved or much improved at the end of treatment. The findings with regard to transfer of learning were variable. In three patients, including the one who failed to improve, reduction in GSR closely followed the course of systematic desensitization, suggesting a close correspondence between imagining a scene during desensitization and in the test situation. However, one patient exhibited a delay and another an almost total lack of transfer during most of the treatment course. Improvement in objective performance lagged behind progress in desensitization in three out of four patients, and the patient who showed no lag in objective performance exhibited no transfer to the test items.

The findings of this study appear to be discrepant with those of

Rachman. Clearly differences in the investigations could account for this. Agras was studying patients whose phobias might be more refractory to treatment than the fears of 'normal' volunteers. Agras points out that immediate testing by exposure to the actual feared situation in the presence of the therapist may constitute a form of transfer training in itself. He suggests that the variability in reported findings of degree and speed of generalization may be related to such factors as the degree of the patient's dependency on the therapist and the motivation of the therapist. More recently, Agras *et al.* (1968) have demonstrated that praise by the therapist can act as an effective social reinforcer and increase the distance that agoraphobics travel. Finally he concluded that the GSR evoked by imagination of the feared situation did not serve as a useful indicator of actual therapeutic improvement.

The last finding has received some support from Hoenig and Reed (1966) who treated four patients with monosymptomatic phobias by systematic desensitization and employed two different measures to assess outcome. The first involved the measurement of GSR to the key phobic word inserted in a word association test, imagination of the phobic stimulus, and presentation of the real phobic stimulus. The other method of assessment was the more conventional clinical assessment relying largely on verbal reports from patients and relatives. Treatment and clinical assessments were carried out without knowledge of the physiological measurements. The results of this study showed that there could be considerable variance between clinical assessment and changes in GSR. There was more agreement between clinical assessment and physiological response to the verbal than to imagined or real stimuli.

There is considerable evidence that autonomic measures can reflect the behavioural manifestations and subjective feelings of anxiety. To the extent that they provide an additional source of information for the difficult task of assessing changes in emotional state, they may prove to be of clinical and prognostic value (Lader *et al.*, 1967; Gelder and Mathews, 1968; Kelly and Walter, 1968). However, expensive and elaborate apparatus is required and evaluation of tracings presents considerable difficulties (Martin, I., 1960; Martin, B., 1961, 1969; Venables and Martin, 1967). Furthermore, correlations are not always

high for either within subject or between subject recordings of autonomic measures and clinical ratings. Where discrepancies exist the
therapist is likely to join with his patient in giving priority to overt
behaviour and subjective experience rather than some physiological
variable. There is great difficulty in the selection, measurement and
interpretation of psycho-physiological variables as a measure of clinical anxiety because of uncertainty concerning the degree of response
specificity and the intercorrelation between different autonomic
variables.

The problem of achieving transfer of systematic desensitization to
real life situations has received further attention in an investigation
conducted by Cooke (1966) which compared desensitization in
imagination and real life in high and low general anxiety subjects.
Twelve female volunteers with an excessive fear of rats were divided
into high and low anxiety groups on the basis of their scores on an
emotionality scale. Two subjects from each group were randomly
allocated to one of three procedures, desensitization to real life stimuli
or imagined stimuli or no-treatment control. The experimental groups
received four treatment sessions. All subjects were assessed before and
five days after treatment on an avoidance test, fear ratings, a questionnaire yielding a general fear and a rat-fear score, and on the emotionality scale. Therapy was conducted by two clinical psychologists and
ratings were made by three independent judges. All ratings of specific
fear improved significantly in the two experimental groups, and slightly more in the direct treatment group. The original level of general
anxiety did not discriminate between the number of items completed
or outcome of direct training. With desensitization in imagination,
low-anxiety subjects completed significantly more items in treatment
than high-anxiety subjects, yet the latter showed a greater reduction in
specific fear of rats. The finding that high-anxiety individuals fared as
well as low-anxiety ones is at variance with the previously cited studies
with psychiatric patients and Paul's investigation of volunteers with
fear of public speaking. In view of the small number of subjects studied
by Cooke, this point requires further elucidation. However, the bulk
of evidence already available suggests that there is no exact correlation
between progress in systematic desensitization in the treatment situation and the person's behaviour in the outside world. Obviously a

large number of variables influence this and it would be naïve to expect that they would all be subsumed under a general emotionality scale.

A further study related to the differential effects of imagined and actual exposure in desensitization has been reported by Garfield *et al.* (1967) in a pilot investigation of seven volunteers with a snake phobia. They were randomly allocated to one of two groups. Four subjects received eight sessions of desensitization in imagination and three were given four *in vivo* sessions in addition to eight imaginal sessions. Outcome was measured by performance in an avoidance test before and after treatment. All subjects improved significantly, but those who received *in vivo* training in addition not surprisingly fared significantly better. Obviously the limitations of such a pilot study allow no firm conclusions to be drawn, but the expectation that a combination of real life and imaginal desensitization is superior to imagination alone receives support. However, Barlow *et al.* (1969) have carried out a direct comparison between desensitization in imagination and *in vivo* in twenty college students with a fear of snakes. Both treatment methods included relaxation and graded presentation of heirarchy items. *In vivo* desensitization was significantly better than imaginal as measured by avoidance test and GSR. Imaginal desensitization only reduced GSRs to imagined stimuli.

As yet there are few studies of the vicarious desensitization of fears. Bandura *et al.* (1967) studied forty-eight children who exhibited marked avoidance behaviour in the presence of dogs. They were allocated to one of four groups. The first group participated in 'modelling sessions' in which they observed a 'fearless peer model' engaged in progressively larger and closer interactions with a dog within a 'pleasurable context' of a party. The second group were submitted to the same procedure in a neutral context; the third group observed the dog in the pleasurable context but without the peer model (controlling for exposure to the dog), whilst the fourth group engaged in pleasurable activities without exposure to the dog or the peer model. All groups showed a reduction in avoidance behaviour to the test dog and an unfamiliar dog one month later, but both modelling procedures led to significantly greater and more stable improvement. The 'pleasurable context' added little to the outcome.

In a further controlled study Bandura and Menlove (1968) compared the effects of watching films of a single model with one dog and watching films of several models with a variety of dogs on the reduction of fear and avoidance of dogs in forty-eight three- to five-year-old children. Although there was a significant reduction in fear ratings in treated as opposed to untreated controls immediately after treatment, the expected superiority of the multiple modelling procedure, assessed by the criterion response of handling the dog, was only evident at one month follow-up. Immediately after treatment there was no difference in the proportion able to perform the criterion response between either treated or untreated groups. Another finding of interest (consistent with the findings of systematic desensitization in imagination) was that 'high emotional proneness', measured by a questionnaire completed by the parent, impaired the reduction of anxiety of dogs by modelling procedures.

Ritter (1968) compared the efficacy of observation of fearless model behaviour ('vicarious desensitization') with a combination of observation and opportunity to touch the phobic object or the model during the period of observation. Forty-four pre-adolescent children with a fear of snakes were allocated to one of the two treatment procedures or a no-treatment control group. Treatment consisted of two thirty-five-minute sessions. As expected, both treatments resulted in a significant reduction in avoidance behaviour in the post treatment avoidance test, but the combined procedure (80 per cent able to perform criterion response) was superior to the vicarious procedure alone (53·3 per cent). The controls showed no improvement. Changes in subjective reports of anxiety while performing the avoidance tasks also changed in the expected direction but did not reach a significant level.

Bandura *et al.* (1968) investigated the comparative efficacy of modelling and desensitization in the treatment of adolescents and adults with a fear of snakes. Forty-five subjects were matched according to their behaviour in an avoidance test and allocated to one of four groups. The first observed a film showing adults and children behaving in a fearless manner in progressively more anxiety-evoking situations. The subjects were relaxed and able to control their rate of exposure to the film. The second group observed live models and gradually participated in approaching and handling the snake themselves. The third received systematic desensitization in imagination.

Experimental studies of conditioning in enuresis

The fourth were a no-treatment control group who only participated in the behavioural interview assessments. The results showed that the second procedure (live modelling combined with guided participation) was the most effective. Symbolic modelling (Group 1) and systematic desensitization (Group 3) caused substantial reductions in avoidance behaviour, while the control group was unchanged. All those who had failed the terminal approach performance test were then given live modelling with participation. Snake phobic behaviour was successfully extinguished within a few brief sessions in all subjects. In addition, this method also produced the largest decrease in self-rated anxiety and the most generalization in diminishing social and other fears.

O'Neill and Howell (1969) compared the effects of systematic desensitization to imagined scenes, photographs and live modelling without participation in volunteer snake phobics. All three methods produced significant improvement and there was no significant difference between them.

All these studies suggest that the more realistic the presentation and the greater the degree of participation of subject and model, the more effective is the treatment.

Experimental studies of conditioning in enuresis

In a monograph Lovibond (1964) presents a comprehensive review of the literature on enuresis and reports the results of his own experimental studies with animals and enuretic children. Some of this work has already been discussed in previous chapters. Although both the aetiology and theoretical basis of conditioning therapy of enuresis are still disputed, there is evidence that Mowrer's, Crosby's and Lovibond's twin-signal methods can lead to arrest of the condition without causing adverse psychological reactions. It will be remembered that Lovibond favoured a conditioned avoidance paradigm rather than classical conditioning. He conducted a field study to compare the efficacy of the three types of treatment in thirty-six children randomly allocated to one of the three procedures. Treatment was continued to a criterion response of approximately fourteen consecutive dry nights. For those children who had completed seven dry nights, fluid intake was increased. Treatment was considered to have failed if the criterion had not been achieved after fifty reinforcements. As predicted, the twin-signal was the most successful method as judged by the number of reinforcements required to attain the criterion. However, the relapse rate was high (four to five children in each group) and Lovibond's hypothesis that the twin-signal would lead to greater resistance to extinction was not supported. But the fact that treatment could succeed without necessarily awakening the child and the amount of urine excreted gradually decreased during the course of treatment, is considered by Lovibond to support the hypothesis that stimulation arising from the act of micturition becomes the conditioned avoidance stimulus.

Lovibond conducted further experiments focused mainly on the problem of relapse. It had already been shown that high levels of avoidance behaviour could be established by the administration of the UCS alone not contingent on any behaviour (Sidman *et al.*, 1957). Using rats, Lovibond found that 'free shocks' helped to maintain the avoidance response during extinction trials and after. He then investigated the effect of administering 'false alarms' with the Mowrer and twin-signal methods. Twenty enuretic children were matched for age, sex and frequency of bedwetting and randomly allocated to either the Mowrer or twin-signal apparatus. Half the children in each treatment received twelve 'false alarms' from the bell or hooter on twelve consecutive nights following the first two dry nights. Those who did not achieve the success criterion of fourteen dry nights were given random alternations of false alarms and correct signalling for the remainder of the treatment period. In fact all children reached the required criterion and there were negligible differences between the treatment groups as regards the median number of trials required to produce initial arrest, which was less than that required in the previous experiment. Consistent with expectations, the number relapsing during the first three months was lower in the false alarm group than the standard group, but the difference was insignificant. But the final relapse rate (over three to twenty-four months) in the false alarm treatment (50 per cent) was nearly as high as with the standard procedure (60 per cent). Slightly greater resistance to extinction was found with the Mowrer apparatus.

Lovibond's findings so far have suggested that the twin-signal tends to produce a more rapid initial arrest than the Mowrer apparatus, but the latter leads to greater resistance to extinction. He pointed out that this difference in treatment outcome may be due to two differences in the treatment procedures, namely stimulus duration and intensity. The more rapid acquisition with the twin-signal might be due to the provision of escape training rather than the intensity of its aversive hooter stimulus, while the continuing relatively weaker stimulus in the Mowrer instrument may be responsible for the greater resistance to extinction. Thus an apparatus which provided an initial strong stimulus followed by a weaker stimulus of longer duration would combine the virtues of both instruments. Lovibond also considered the alternative hypothesis that the superiority of the twin-signal method in acquisition might be due to its more intensive aversive stimulus rather than its provision for escape training. This would be predicted on theoretical grounds if the conditioning treatment consisted of passive avoidance learning in which continence is part of an unconditioned response rather than a conditioned response. In this case the important variables influencing its acquisition would be the intensity and duration of the aversive stimulus.

In an attempt to elucidate this problem, Lovibond carried out an investigation on rats and another with enuretic children. The animal study suggested that for the establishment of a passive avoidance response the critical variable was the intensity of the shock rather than its pattern or duration, whereas resistance to extinction was greater when weak initial shocks of relatively long duration had been given. The study of enuretics involved twenty-four subjects allocated to either the Mowrer instrument (weak continuous stimulation) or a modified twin-signal consisting of a brief intense stimulus followed by a weaker stimulus of longer duration. Although no significant differences were obtained, the modified apparatus produced slightly quicker acquisition and Mowrer's instrument led to slightly greater resistance to extinction.

Thus the three field experiments tentatively but consistently suggest that a short intense stimulus produces more rapid acquisition and less resistance to extinction, irrespective of whether or not it is followed by a longer less intense stimulus or combined with false alarms. Lovibond reports two further investigations, one with rats and one with enuretics to test the theoretical prediction that intermittent reinforcement would increase the resistance to extinction of a passive avoidance response. The standard avoidance treatment procedure employs continuous reinforcement and would be expected to be less efficient in this respect. The rat experiment bore out this expectation. Acquisition of a passive avoidance response using intermittent strong shock (50 per cent of trials randomly administered) was comparable to that obtained with continuous weak reinforcement. Partial reinforcement with weak or variable-strength shock resulted in significantly poorer acquisition. All three intermittent procedures produced significantly greater resistance to extinction than the continuous weak reinforcement procedure. Significantly greater resistance to extinction was obtained with intermittent strong shocks than with intermittent weak shocks.

In a study of sixteen enuretic children treated with the standard twin-signal instrument, parents were provided with a random alternation reinforcement schedule and instructed to switch off the apparatus when non-reinforcement was scheduled. For comparative purposes, results of the three previous experiments with enuretics were used. Over a twelve-month period, only three children (19 per cent) relapsed, in comparison with 35 per cent and 44 per cent with complete reinforcement with the Mowrer and twin-signal methods. However, the diminution in relapse rate with partial reinforcement did not reach statistical significance.

The main criticism of Lovibond's work is that the enuretic children studied formed a rather selected sample. Although his results are indecisive, the studies offer an excellent example of the systematic investigation of problems associated with a particular behavioural anomaly and provide a stimulating source for further research.

Young and Turner (1965), in a study referred to in the previous chapter, tested the hypothesis that stimulant drugs facilitate the process of conditioning (see Eysenck, 1957; Franks and Trouton, 1958). The Eastleigh buzzer and pad apparatus alone was employed in the treatment of 105 children, in another eighty-four children it was combined with dexamphetamine sulphate 5–15 mg, and a third group of 110 children received methylamphetamine hydrochloride 2·5–7·5 mg. The failure rate was similar in all three groups, but the two drug groups responded significantly faster than the group with the apparatus alone, and dexamphetamine was significantly superior to methylamphetamine. Unfortunately, the relapse rate during an extended follow-up period (ranging from nine months to five years) of 142 children (Turner and Young, 1966) revealed a significantly higher relapse rate in the dexamphetamine group (75·6 per cent) than in the methylamphetamine group (43 per cent), which in turn was significantly more than in the non-drug group (31·7 per cent). Thus the more rapid development of continence associated with the addition of drugs led to a drastic relapse rate. This study raises many questions. In particular it would be of interest to know whether a gradual withdrawal of drugs would reduce the high relapse rate.

In a theoretical study to test Eysenck's hypothesis concerning the relationship between introversion and speed of conditionability, Young (1965) administered the Junior Maudsley Personality Inventory (Furneaux and Gibson, 1961) to seventy-nine enuretic children prior to their receiving treatment. A significantly higher relapse rate was found in extraverted than in introverted children, thus demonstrating a relationship between extraversion and rapid extinction.

Aversion therapy

There is naturally a strong reluctance on the part of clinicians to use punishment as a form of treatment for patients, so that despite its long and traditional usage by parents, teachers and society, attempts have been made to delineate accurately the type of patient and kind of disorder which will respond to aversion therapy and the indications for its use. These will be determined by the usual criteria for assessing any therapeutic procedure, namely the wishes of the patient, its efficacy, undesirable side effects, the availability of other treatments, and the likely course of the disorder if left untreated. Research in this direction has been focused on the search for prognostic variables, improving the efficacy of treatment procedures and investigating whether aversive stimulation is a necessary ingredient of successful treatment.

Morgenstern *et al.* (1965) administered a battery of nine psychological tests to nineteen patients who requested treatment for transvestism. Six failed to attend for treatment, six improved significantly after treatment and seven stopped cross-dressing altogether. Studying these three outcome groups separately, the 'cured' group differed from the others in being significantly less neurotic (N score of MP1), showing a better response to a verbal conditioning procedure, and less femininity on a masculinity–femininity scale. The cured group also tended to be more intelligent, less anxious and less introverted, but these did not reach statistical significance. It is of interest that facility of eyeblink conditioning did not appear relevant to outcome whereas verbal conditioning did. The authors tentatively suggested that an operant form of conditioning is involved in aversion therapy. One could also speculate that language plays a significant part in this.

It will be remembered that Feldman and MacCulloch argued that avoidance learning was likely to be more effective than classical conditioning in aversion therapy and adopted this method for the treatment of homosexuality which was described in chapter 4. MacCulloch *et al.* (1965) investigated the latency of avoidance responses and pulse-rate changes following the presentation of photographs of nude males during the treatment of four patients. Their findings indicated that in those patients who improved with treatment there was a gradual decrease in avoidance-response latency, suggesting that therapeutic success was related to specific learning. In patients who did not improve with treatment decrease in response latency was not observed. Similarly, in one patient who responded to treatment a conditioned response of increased pulse rate was established, whereas no such response occurred in a patient who failed to respond to treatment.

Marks and Gelder (1967) have reported a detailed study of the process of electric aversion therapy administered to three transvestites and two fetishists. It will be recalled that treatment was directed to both overt behaviour and fantasy. Changes in treatment were evaluated by clinical assessment, occurrence of penile erections by a penis transducer (see Bancroft *et al.*, 1966), and change in attitudes on semantic differential scales (Marks, 1965; Marks and Sartorius, 1968). Erections during the fantasy or execution of deviant behaviour were extinguished during treatment. However, little generalization occurred so that it was necessary to establish aversion to each particular garment in turn. Erections to normal heterosexual stimuli were not affected by the treatment, and attitudes changed in the expected direction only to the clothes to which treatment had been directed.

When aversion to fantasies was being established, it was found that the time taken by the patient to imagine the item gradually lengthened until finally it was impossible to fantasy it. Before treatment, erections often preceded the fantasy; after treatment no erections occurred. This gradual increase in latency and decrease in erections only occurred when aversive stimuli were given. Marks (1968a) suggests that this is an internal conditioned avoidance response rather than a voluntary response, and considers it to be an example of experimental repression. Only some patients showed clinical evidence of anxiety while repression developed, and physiological measures of anxiety were not always present. Many patients showed depression, anxiety or irritability during the course of treatment. One patient complained of long-lasting symptoms of irritability and lack of creative ability, which lasted for six months after discharge from hospital and subsided when the patient partially relapsed into fetishist activity. Obviously this may be an example of symptom substitution in which removal of one symptom, fetishism, was replaced by irritability. However, another possible explanation is that the deviant sexual drive had not been completely eliminated. Patients who had lost their deviant sexual feelings showed improvement in other spheres of life, whereas depression and irritability may have occurred before or during treatment or on relapse. One patient who attempted suicide when he relapsed into his deviant behaviour had previously developed depressive symptoms after cross-dressing. It does not appear that symptom substitution is a special risk of aversion therapy, but patients can develop psychological reactions during the course of treatment, as well as when untreated, which may require treatment.

Madill *et al.* (1966) described a clinical investigation of aversion therapy with drug-induced apnoea in the treatment of alcoholism. They wished to determine whether their method fulfilled the requirements of classical conditioning; whether a conditioned emotional response was established to alcohol; whether avoidance responses to alcohol developed and whether clinical improvement took place. Forty-five alcoholic patients were randomly allocated to one of three groups: conditioning (CS and UCS); pseudoconditioning (UCS alone); and control (CS alone). Each patient was given a few drops of his favourite drink to look at, smell and taste. This procedure was repeated three times. Then the conditioning group were given a drink again within ten seconds of the onset of the UCS (succinylcholine apnoea), while apnoea was induced in the pseudoconditioning group without a further presentation of alcohol. After this, all three groups were presented with alcohol alone for three trials. A continuous record of GSR, respiratory and pulse rates, muscle tension and electro-cardiogram were made, and the length of apnoea and speed of onset and intensity of fear were observed. The patients' drinking and general behaviour were assessed three months before and three months after treatment.

The onset of apnoea rather than its duration appeared to be the important determinant of aversion. All groups developed a generalized anxiety response immediately after treatment. It was quicker and more intense in the conditioning and pseudoconditioning groups than in the control group, but this was not statistically significant. However, generalized avoidance responses to alcohol were found significantly more frequently in the two treated groups. The amount of alcohol drunk decreased significantly in the two treatment groups and drinking less often took place at the haunts favoured before treatment. However, there was no significant difference in the reduction of craving or number of days abstinent between the three groups.

The over-all results of treatment were poor, but it is only fair to add that the patients selected for treatment were likely to have had a poor response to any treatment. The authors concluded that although the method successfully produced conditioned aversive emotional responses, they were not sufficient to alter drinking behaviour. An unexpected finding in the study was the lack of difference between conditioning and 'pseudoconditioning'. At first sight this might suggest that none of the changes following treatment could be attributed to conditioning by contiguity. However, as the authors point out, conditioning may still have taken place in the pseudoconditioning group because of the presentation of alcohol three times in the treatment situation before the induction of apnoea. The fear evoked by this procedure could become associated with alcohol. Certainly patients would be aware that they had been subjected to a frightening experience because they were alcoholics. However, the important point which emerges from this investigation is that the acquisition of conditioned aversive emotional responses is not itself sufficient to alter operant behaviour. The authors drew attention to experimental results showing that punishment may be ineffective in eliminating behaviour established by punishment (see Holz and Azrin, 1961; Solomon, 1967). Furthermore, the alcoholic may drink in order to reduce anxiety and tension. In these patients, aversion therapy may add a specific anxiety to alcohol to their generalized anxiety, thus producing a 'double avoidance situation'. In view of the poor results and these theoretical considerations a more complete treatment programme is advocated.

Blake's studies (1965, 1967) are relevant in this connexion. It will be recalled that he compared the efficacy of a combination of relaxation and aversion therapy with aversion therapy alone in the treatment of alcoholics. The rationale for employing the combined treatment lay in the suggestion put forward by Eysenck (1960a) that conditioned aversion will not persist if the drive (anxiety) motivating the drinking remains unchanged. The patients in Blake's relaxation-aversion group were first trained in relaxation and instructed to use it to reduce tension occurring in everyday life. After an average of twelve sessions of relaxation training they were submitted to an escape-learning procedure with electric shock. The control group, matched for age, sex, social class, intelligence, chronicity of alcoholism, and psychiatric diagnosis, received aversion therapy only. At twelve months follow-up, 59 per cent of the experimental group and 50 per cent of the controls were rated as either abstinent or improved. The difference was not statistically significant.

One weakness of this study, pointed out by Blake, was that the hypothesis was not tested rigorously because subjects were not selected on the basis of the presence or absence of 'neurotic anxiety'. But apart from this, it is doubtful whether training in relaxation alone is an efficient method of reducing anxiety. Systematic desensitization to specific anxiety-provoking situations is likely to be more effective. Finally, it is difficult to understand why a 'motivational arousal' procedure, aimed at increasing the patients' motivation for treatment by instructing them to think about their drinking and associated problems, was carried out under relaxation.

Specific Processes

Operant conditioning

Studies in this area have concentrated mainly on the problem of demonstrating that changes in behaviour following operant conditioning are due to response-contingent reinforcements. Most of these studies have used psychotic patients as subjects and immediate therapeutic benefit was not always the main aim.

Several investigations have demonstrated that verbal behaviour can be influenced in the expected direction by means of contingent reinforcement. Ayllon and Haughton (1964) reported on an extensive study of three psychotic patients with delusions. Nurses first recorded a baseline measurement of the frequency of 'sick' verbal behaviour in which delusions were expressed and then ascertained the effect of reinforcement and omission of reinforcement on its frequency. Reward of psychotic verbal behaviour increased its frequency while omission of reward decreased it. Reversing the reinforcement schedule produced the opposite effect. Ullmann *et al.* (1965) selected for differential reinforcement 'sick talk' versus 'healthy talk' during a twenty-minute structured interview. The subjects were sixty male chronic schizophrenic patients who were assigned to one of three procedures. In the first, sick talk was reinforced; in the second, healthy talk was reinforced; and in the third, plural nouns were reinforced. Reinforcement consisted of the experimenter smiling, nodding and saying encouragingly 'mmh-hmm'. The results indicated that sick talk decreased in the group rewarded for healthy talk and increased in the other two groups.

Wilson and Walters (1966) compared the efficacy of two different procedures in increasing the amount of speech in near-mute schizophrenics. Four patients were exposed to a talkative model and received reinforcement with pennies when they talked about scenes depicted on slides they were shown. Another four patients were treated in the same way, except that they were not given contingent reinforcements. A third group of four patients were shown the slides but had no talkative model or contingent reinforcement. (All three groups received the same amount of money but in the non-reinforced groups it was given after the treatment session.) In the second stage of the experiment all the subjects were submitted to the model-plus-contingent-reinforcement situation. Increase in speech occurred in the first two groups and

192

was more marked in the model-plus-contingent-reinforcement treatment. Introduction of this procedure to all subjects in the second phase led to significant improvement in all groups.

Ayllon and Azrin (1965) conducted six related experiments over a period of almost three years in an attempt to evaluate the reinforcing effects of token economies described in chapter 4. In each experiment the patient served as his own control. After measurement of response frequency under one reinforcement schedule, the schedule was reversed and then finally reinstated again. Results showed that the tokens were effective in changing voluntary-task choices from initially preferred to non-preferred tasks, while non-contingent administration of tokens led to a decrease in task attendance and removal of tokens from the programme led to a significant decline in task performance. The contingencies could be established by oral or by written instructions from the staff.

In another study previously described, Ayllon and Azrin (1964) investigated the relative contributions of verbal instruction and positive reinforcement in getting patients to collect their eating utensils before entering the hospital canteen. Eighteen female patients, mainly schizophrenics, were studied. If they performed the target behaviour they were rewarded with extra food. Only a slight improvement occurred, mainly because few patients performed any of the target behaviour before treatment started. After the patients were told that they would be rewarded each time they came into the canteen with their utensils, there was a dramatic increase in the desired behaviour. In an attempt to discover whether verbal instructions alone would produce the desired behaviour, a second experiment was conducted on a similar sample of patients. They were given the same instructions as in the previous study, but were not given extra food. But if they did not pick up the cutlery, they were made to wait before entering the canteen. With this procedure the target behaviour increased to between 40–70 per cent. However, when extra food was given as a reward, this figure rose to between 90 per cent and 100 per cent. Ayllon and Azrin concluded that both verbal instructions and positive reinforcement can contribute to the establishment of target behaviour.

A number of studies have attempted to tackle directly the problem of attaining the generalization of effects achieved in the experimental setting to the outside world. Ullmann *et al.* (1964) were able to induce a significant increase in common associations in a word-association test given to schizophrenics, but failed to obtain generalization to common responses to drawings of people. Michenbaum (1966) showed that contingent social reinforcement of abstract thinking in a proverbs test in schizophrenics produced significant improvement which generalized also to a new but related conceptual task.

On the assumption that an increase in emotional expression would improve interpersonal relationships in group therapy, Ullmann *et al.* (1961a and b) employed a verbal conditioning technique in which emotional words used in telling a story were socially reinforced. The patients' behaviour in the group was then reassessed by an independent therapist. In one study the experimental group showed the expected improvement in interpersonal relationships in the group setting, but in the second study the results were equivocal.

In assessing operant conditioning, there is impressive experimental evidence that observed changes in verbal and non-verbal behaviour in psychotic patients following operant conditioning depend upon contingent application of primary and secondary reinforcement. Operant techniques have only been systematically studied in human subjects during the last twenty years, and most investigations have been experimental in nature rather than therapeutically oriented until the recent studies of token economy programmes. Research needs to be directed towards extending changes produced in the experimental setting to everyday life. Psychologists should also realize that attempts to account for all behaviour disorders in terms of some aspect of verbal and non-verbal operant conditioning may well prove to be a gross oversimplification.

In summary, it should be said that one of the most impressive aspects of behaviour therapy, considering its short existence, is the amount of research it has stimulated and the willingness of behaviourists to examine critically their basic assumptions and seek empirical evidence of therapeutic efficacy. One should not lose sight of this objectivity because of the tendency of some to devote energy to intemperate attacks on other forms of treatment. There is a considerable body of evidence showing that specific behaviour therapy techniques can modify some abnormal behaviour. This empirical evidence is consistent with the principles from which the treatments derive but there is a lack of conclusive knowledge as to how they work. At the same time research work has often produced findings which pose new questions and problems requiring further investigation.

It appears that the combination of graduated exposure and relaxation are the most important factors in systematic desensitization and this is the main evidence in support of a counterconditioning process. Systematic desensitization procedures also afford an opportunity for extinction and habituation to occur and these may contribute to therapeutic efficacy. There is also some evidence that the combination of desensitization in imagination and practical retraining is superior to systematic desensitization alone. Consistent with this is the evidence that symbolic modelling and desensitization are inferior to live modelling with participation.

It must be remembered that the majority of studies of systematic desensitization and modelling have been conducted with volunteer subjects rather than with psychiatric patients so that these findings cannot automatically be extended to the latter without replication of the findings in such a population. Other methods of treatment have not been as intensively and widely investigated but some interesting findings begin to emerge. In aversion therapy, there is evidence that conditioned emotional and avoidance responses are established.

Chapter 7

Current Research II: Cognition and Non-Specific Processes of Psychological Treatment

A wide variety of psychological treatments claim some degree of success with certain patients, despite the fact that they are based on different theoretical formulations. This suggests that there are one or more variables common to all types of therapy which are responsible for therapeutic change, and research is required to identify them. Behaviour therapists postulate that learning processes are the critical factor and have accumulated evidence in support of this. Psychodynamic theory emphasizes the attainment of emotional insight and the experience of a therapeutic relationship as the necessary conditions of therapeutic change. It is possible that the two approaches differ only in terminology, or also in their theoretical formulation or also in their therapeutic procedures. Several attempts have been made to find common ground between learning theory and psychoanalytic theory.

The theoretical account of the process of psychotherapy includes the gaining of insight into the unconscious conflicts and defence mechanisms which constitute the symptoms and personality disturbance, their resolution or modification, and maturation of the ego and the development of mature patterns of behaviour. Insight is obtained through the process of exploration and interpretation of free associations and the transference reaction and resistances. Resolution of conflict and modification of defence mechanisms proceed via their repetitive evocation (working through) and the realization that the anxieties are of historical interest rather than of current significance (reality testing). Maturation of the ego and adaptive patterns of behaviour are expected to result from the combination of the removal of defensive stratagems and the experience of relating to a therapist who avoids either being manoeuvred into or spontaneously adopting a role which will perpetuate the patient's maladaptive responses.

Shoben (1949) has suggested that all psychotherapeutic procedures involve three interrelated psychological processes.

First, the lifting of repression and development of insight through the symbolic reinstating of the stimuli for anxiety; second, the diminution of anxiety by counter-conditioning through the attachment of the stimuli for anxiety to the comfort reaction made to the therapeutic relationship; and third, the process of re-education through the therapist's helping the patient to formulate rational goals and behavioural methods for attaining them.

Shoben warns that this description leans on plausible hypotheses and tenuous analogies, but it does offer a persuasive account of the theory and method of psychotherapy in learning terms. Dollard and Miller (1950) also emphasize the importance of lifting repression by identifying and labelling the unconscious anxiety-evoking cues as the first stage in psychotherapy. The permissiveness of the therapist encourages the patient to experience the anxiety cues without any punishing consequences, so that they are gradually extinguished.

It can be seen that it is quite possible to rephrase the postulated processes of psychotherapy in learning terms. Psychodynamic theorists differ in the emphasis they attach to insight and relationship factors as the agents of therapeutic change, but the importance of the relationship has received increasing recognition. If we consider the actual method of psychotherapy, with its exploration of feelings and relationships, it will be seen that anxiety cues may be exposed and avoidance responses can be elicited. The special characteristics of the therapeutic relationship will provide an opportunity for extinction or counterconditioning. In addition the psychotherapist can serve as a model for imitation, vicarious extinction, and the source of positive and negative reinforcement for operant conditioning. Because psychotherapy could provide an opportunity for the full range of learning procedures used by behaviour therapists, the latter can account for the successes of psychotherapy in terms of learning principles. They would add that psychotherapy is an elaborate and haphazard way of conducting behaviour therapy, and that their own strategy of treatment creates a more systematic and efficient learning situation for the modification of unwanted behaviour. A possible demonstration of the role of counterconditioning in psychotherapy is provided by Wilson and Smith (1968) in which two patients were encouraged to free associate while maintaining deep muscular relaxation. For this type of patient the amount of improvement apparently obtained in a small number of sessions is impressive. Counter-conditioning may have been the important therapeutic process but obviously further investigation is required before any conclusions can be drawn.

Many workers have stressed the importance of learning processes in psychotherapy (e.g. Mowrer, 1950; Bandura, 1961; Alexander, 1963; Piers and Piers, 1965; Marks and Gelder, 1966). Some have regarded it as basically a verbal interaction process subject to verbal conditioning (e.g. Krasner, 1958; Kanfer, 1961), but others have emphasized the difference between verbal conditioning and psychotherapy, emphasizing the more complex emotional changes in the latter (e.g. Luborsky and Strupp, 1962).

Probably no one would deny that verbal conditioning can occur even in 'non-directive' psychotherapy. (See, for example, the study of Truax, 1966b, which is discussed on p. 208). Whether this is welcomed and thought of as desirable by the theorist or clinician will depend on his views as to its efficacy in achieving the goals of therapy. The psychotherapist expects change in behaviour to occur in the patient as a result of new ways of feeling and thinking which emerge in the treatment situation in which the method of communication is largely verbal.[1] It is therefore expected that the new kinds of subjective experience occurring in treatment will modify experience and behaviour outside of treatment. If it is conceptualized as verbal conditioning, it must be assumed that modification of verbal behaviour can generate changes in other kinds of behaviour (see Metzner, 1961; Krasner, 1963, 1965). Research in this area has been very limited, but obviously the extensive use of language in education suggests that its efficacy is assumed. In normal children experimental studies have demonstrated

1. This obviously imposes some restrictions on the types of patients who can be treated by psychotherapy. Friedman (1966b) reports the successful treatment of a dog phobia in a deaf mute by systematic desensitization with graduated presentation of photographs of dogs to the patient under methohexitone relaxation. Leaving aside theoretical considerations, it would be difficult to imagine such a patient in psychotherapy.

a direct transfer from verbal to non-verbal behaviour (e.g. Lovaas, 1961, 1964). Brodsky (1967) investigated this problem in two asocial retarded institutionalized adolescents. In one girl the imitation of social behaviour in a structured setting was reinforced. This led to an increase in social behaviour in treatment which generalized to a play-ground setting, and subsequently to verbal behaviour in interviews. The second patient was rewarded for uttering social statements in interviews. Although a verbal conditioning effect was obtained, there was no generalization to the structured setting or to social behaviour in the playground. No conclusions can be drawn from such a limited investigation, but clearly transfer from verbal to non-verbal behaviour is not always automatic. Luria (1961) has presented some evidence suggesting that verbal behaviour effectively controls non-verbal behaviour only when the external verbal command has been 'internalized'.

There is well-established evidence that systematic changes in verbal behaviour occur in verbal conditioning analogues of psychotherapy (Greenspoon, 1962) and in psychotherapy (see Bandura, 1961; Frank, 1961). However, there is little evidence for the generalization of such effects from the therapeutic situation to other behaviours (Zax and Klein, 1960; Kanfer, 1961; Greenspoon, 1962). Clearly related to this problem is the role of insight in therapy. It is one of the main goals of various types of psychotherapy and psychoanalysis (e.g. Fenichel, 1946; Rogers, 1951; Sullivan, 1953). It is postulated that self-knowledge of the reasons for his behaviour will allow the patient to modify it. In learning terms, discrimination learning takes place as the cues are uncovered and maladaptive responses extinguished. The elimination of anxiety responses in insight (and possibly implosive) therapy requires a knowledge of how they were acquired. In most forms of behaviour therapy, on the other hand, the tendency is to bypass cognitive processes (see London, 1964, for a comparison of 'insight' and 'action' therapy).

Many therapists have questioned the importance of 'insight' in bringing about behaviour change. Alexander and French (1946), for instance, consider that insight is the result rather than a precondition of change. Hobbs (1962) concluded that personality change can occur independently of insight which is sometimes a by-product of such change. Experimental evidence on this subject is not clearcut. Heap and Sipprelle (1966) found that insight was unrelated to the extinction of an operant verbal response, whereas Cole and Sipprelle (1967) demonstrated that awareness was positively related to the extinction of a classical GSR response. As already described, awareness can influence the operant conditioning of patients. Bandura (1969) includes an excellent review of experimental studies of the relationship between awareness and behavioural change, and concludes that awareness is a powerful facilitative factor but may not be a necessary or sufficient condition for classical or instrumental conditioning. Obviously the role of insight is a complex one. It is certainly not warranted to consider that it can always modify behaviour. It is necessary to study which kind of symptoms in what type of situation are susceptible to change through insight.

The origin and type of symptom are probably relevant in this regard. An example of the importance of the origin of a particular symptom is provided by Bridger and Mandel's study previously described, in which one group of subjects received a strong electric shock following a CS, while the other group were warned that they would receive a shock following the CS but in fact never received it. Both groups showed GSR responses to the CS. However, when the electrodes were removed and the subjects informed that they would not be shocked, there was immediate extinction in the verbally threatened group but not in the group who had received the shock. It appears that verbal instructions have less influence on conditioned responses acquired through physical trauma. Bridger and Mandel suggest that verbal manipulation may be ineffective for patients whose phobias developed as a result of physical trauma and it may be necessary for them to experience extinction trials without it. In Pavlovian terms, modification of behaviour acquired through the 'first signalling system' (autonomic) requires the submission of this system to new experiences; whereas in cases where the 'second signalling system' (speech) is involved alone, it is sufficient to remove subjective expectancy through the medium of language. Furthermore, the lack of effect of verbal instructions with the first group is consistent with the clinical finding that patients with phobias are usually aware that their fears are unrealistic, but this does not reduce their intensity.

201

Both learning and psychodynamic theorists consider that anxiety usually forms the main basis of neurotic disorders and that symptoms are mediated and maintained by the need for anxiety reduction (defence mechanisms). However, there is no evidence that this is the only way that symptoms develop or persist. Some behaviour disorders may result from a lack of opportunity for adequate learning or from maladaptive learning resulting from an inconsistent or unsuitable application of reinforcements. Furthermore, some symptoms may in time become divorced from their original sources of anxiety and may be maintained by secondary reinforcements. A relevant example may be Walton and Mather's (1963) finding that, in obsessive compulsive disorders of recent onset, treatment of the CAD was sufficient, whereas in long-standing cases both the original sources of anxiety and the rituals had to be treated. They argued that the performance of the rituals in the longer standing cases was no longer contingent upon the original anxiety. In addition to maintenance by secondary reinforcement, some disorders, such as involuntary movements and addictions, may become autonomous as a result of biochemical or structural changes associated with their repetitive occurrence. The relative inefficacy of psychotherapy and systematic desensitization in these conditions, and their response to negative practice or aversion therapy, provides some support for the hypothesis that they are not being maintained by anxiety.

Apart from the possibility that some symptoms originally mediated by anxiety may no longer be dependent on it, behaviour therapists should not lose sight of cognitive factors which may be an integral part of some disorders. Valins and Ray (1967) have demonstrated the effect of cognitive reappraisal in reducing fears. The importance of covert thinking and feeling (coverants) in operant conditioning has received attention (Holland and Skinner, 1961; Hefferline, 1962; Staats and Staats, 1963; Homme, 1965) and they are used in operant therapeutic techniques. Verbal instructions have been employed successfully in expediting the establishment of target behaviour (e.g. Ayllon and Azrin, 1964, 1965). Peterson and London (1965) have emphasized the role of cognitive factors in behavioural treatment and considered that the successful treatment in three sessions of a three-year-old with severe constipation was a consequence of the combination of verbal instruction and reinforcement. The importance of concepts and fantasies in the initiation and maintenance of overt behaviour disorders has been recognized in the attention that is directed to them in the more recent aversion therapy procedures. Similarly, the use of emotive imagery as a counterconditioning response and the assumption that desensitization in imagination can transfer to manifest behaviour illustrate that behaviour therapists accept that 'subjective mental experiences' can exert a powerful influence on overt behaviour. Nevertheless, in comparison to the rich diversity and complexity of human language and inner mental experience, the formal use made of them by most behaviour therapy techniques so far must appear trifling and banal. There are historical reasons for this in that behaviour therapy claims to derive from experimental learning theory which is based mainly on animal studies and it has been applied in a clinical setting to disorders in which more sophisticated cognitive approaches have often met with failure or only moderate success.

Some abnormalities of behaviour may be due entirely to faulty attitudes or beliefs and their correction by simple explanation, instruction or demonstration may lead to rapid cures. Unfortunately, it is seldom that a disorder of some duration which leads to referral to a psychiatric clinic will respond to such simple measures. Presumably it is because it is not easily corrected by simple explanation that it has persisted and specialist advice has been sought. But of course, this may also be a result of the complexity of the cognitive disorder which necessitates a more elaborate but still a cognitive approach. A theory which considers cognitive organization pre-eminent in personality development and neurosis has been expounded by Kelly (1955) and provides a basis for the examination of an individual's personal system of constructs (see Bannister and Mair, 1968).

In view of these considerations which we have only been able to outline very briefly, the behaviour therapist should attempt to assess whether the patient's disorder is primarily motor, autonomic or conceptual. Clear-cut cases falling into one category only are rare and one usually finds an admixture of all (e.g. obsessive–compulsive disorders). Despite this, many behaviour therapists tend to regard behaviour therapy as synonymous with systematic desensitization or operant conditioning and there is therefore a tendency to put the patient into a 'theoretical straight-jacket' indiscriminately and more often than not this will lead to the misapplication of behaviour therapy. Lazarus has aptly pointed out the deficiencies of such a narrow approach and advocates a 'broad spectrum behaviour therapy' for complex disorders consisting of a number of behaviour therapy methods in combination. (Lazarus, 1966b; Lazarus and Serber, 1968.) The therapist makes use of learning principles which he applies in an explicit and systematic fashion in his therapeutic plan.

Apart from factors considered to be specific to particular methods of psychological treatment such as insight and learning processes, there are several factors which are operative in most forms of treatment and are therefore labelled 'non-specific'. Included in this category are a number of therapist, patient and interactional variables. The role of suggestion in treatment has received considerable attention and is the main feature of some techniques. However, in many forms of treatment suggestion plays a part even though insight or learning are the main processes thought to be involved. When improvement occurs as a result of suggestion alone, some theorists are unhappy with the outcome because their theory predicts that recovery is unlikely to be maintained. Investigations of physical and psychological treatment attempt to control for suggestion and placebo effects. This is the rationale for double-blind drug trials in which patients receive either a drug or an inert placebo and are assessed without either the patient or doctor knowing which they have received. In many such trials about 30 per cent of subjects receiving the inert substance show significant improvement or deterioration and are referred to as positive and negative placebo reactors respectively. Although changes are more frequently reported in subjective symptoms, objective physiological changes can also occur (Beecher, 1955; Liberman, 1962; Honigfeld, 1964). It has often been assumed that the placebo effect is a function of suggestion, but the correlation between tests of suggestibility and placebo response are not very striking. It seems most likely that placebo reactivity is not a stable personality trait (Liberman, 1964; Shapiro, 1968) but is influenced by the particular clinical and environmental factors operative at the time. It is possible of course to explain a placebo reaction in terms of conditioning in which the placebo is a CS evoking improvement as a result of the patient's previous experience of recovery with medication (see Knowles, 1963). There is some evidence suggesting that high confidence in doctors, favourable attitudes to hospitals and drugs, high levels of discomfort including anxiety and depression, and extraversion are associated with positive placebo reactions (Black, 1966). One important variable in the placebo response is the doctor himself. It has long been recognized that doctors can achieve quite different treatment results although they are using the same drug for the same kinds of patient. The therapist influence may result in a generalized increase or decrease in therapeutic efficacy, but it can also have more subtle effects. Some doctors have been able to obtain a differential effect between an active drug and an inert placebo in their patients in a double-blind trial whereas the patients of other doctors in the same trial consistently showed no difference in response to the active drug and placebo (Uhlenhuth *et al.*, 1959; Joyce, 1962). This provides an elegant demonstration that therapist variables can be more influential than the pharmacological effect of active drugs.

Placebo effects can play a large role in psychological treatment as well as in drug therapy. When a placebo pill is given during the first interview, a significant reduction in subjective symptoms (anxiety and depression) can be manifested at the end of the interview. This symptomatic improvement, as opposed to improved life adjustment, remains stable over the course of time and does not appear to be related to the duration of psychotherapy (Frank, 1961; Frank *et al.*, 1962). In fact some of the improvement takes place early in the interview before the placebo pill is given. The 'placebo effect' can be mediated by the diagnostic interview alone or even by a pill which the patient is told is inert (Park and Covi, 1965). Obviously the expectancy of the patient and aspects of the communication between therapist and patient must be involved. Goldstein (1962, 1968) has emphasized the influence of the patient's expectancy on the outcome of treatment and Friedman (1963) has demonstrated a significant correlation between the patient's expectation of improvement and degree of improvement reported after the first interview. Expectation of improvement can be increased by induction procedures in which the patient is told about the method of psychotherapy and the manner in which it will help him to improve

(Hoehn-Saric *et al.*, 1965). Setting a time limit for the duration of treatment may also have a beneficial influence on outcome (Phillips and Wiener, 1966).

These influences have been conceptualized in terms of hope, faith, suggestion, expectation, and in providing structure and meaning (Frank, 1968). For instance, any interpretations or explanations, whether or not valid, may be beneficial if accepted by the patient because they make his behaviour understandable and therefore less likely to be anxiety evoking. Theoretical formulations of these processes have been couched in terms of conditioning or transference. There is no reason to believe that, whatever the theoretical explanation, these factors will not also be a potent influence in behaviour techniques. Marks *et al.* (1968) have speculated that suggestion may be successful in improving phobias by reducing the patients' anticipatory anxiety and allowing practical retraining to take place. Paul (1966), considered that attention placebo effects (which accounted for about 50 per cent of the improvement in systematic desensitization treatment and nearly 100 per cent of the 'insight therapy') had their influence primarily on attitudes and expectancies rather than on direct modification of emotional reactions.

It is customary clinical practice for behaviour therapists to give an explanation to the patient of how the symptoms were acquired and are being maintained and how learning principles will be used to eliminate them. Furthermore, the patient is usually told about the efficacy of the treatment in which he actively participates, and the therapist's enthusiasm and expectancies may be communicated to the patient.

Lazarus (1968b) conducted a pilot study attempting to evaluate the effects of explanation given prior to desensitization. Out of eight patients treated without preliminary explanation only four improved, whereas five out of six 'similar' patients who were given an explanation of the treatment beforehand showed improvement. In the same paper Lazarus describes an investigation which attempts to assess the contribution of suggestion and structure in behaviour modification. Thirty patients were allocated to one of three forms of treatment. Group 1 received a combination of behaviour therapy methods, group 2 received 'interpretive psychotherapy' and group 3 were administered a structured-suggestion procedure consisting of four phases: examination of salient life experiences; discussion of the meaning of some responses to the incomplete sentence test; discussion of self-actualization concept; visual, auditory and awareness training. The patients in this group were told that they would be promoted from one phase to another on the basis of brief qualifying tests. All groups were informed that treatment would consist of twelve sessions only and that additional therapy, if required, would be available elsewhere. According to a questionnaire all groups showed improvement and no significant differences in outcome between the groups was observed, although there was a tendency for behaviour therapy and structured-suggestion to produce better results than psychotherapy. There are obvious flaws in this investigation which the author himself comments on, but he concludes that a graduated structured-treatment programme which the patient is aware of in advance and in which he can experience a sense of achievement as he completes each stage is likely to enhance therapeutic efficacy. Leitenberg *et al.* (1969) demonstrated that the combination of therapeutic instructions and positive reinforcement by praise significantly improved the efficacy of systematic desensitization in volunteers with a fear of snakes. In a later study (Oliveau *et al.*, 1969), it appeared that therapeutic instructions had a significant effect but that verbal praise given after the successful imagination of hierarchy items did not.

Obviously factors such as suggestion, expectancies of patient and therapist, explanation and structuring will influence and be influenced by the type of relationship that develops between patient and therapist. The importance of the therapeutic relationship has been widely recognized by psychotherapists and relatively ignored by behaviour therapists until recently. Wilson *et al.* (1968) attempted to analyse its effects within a learning framework. There is lack of agreement on its importance, nature, and the critical factors involved (see the discussion by Goldstein *et al.*, 1966). There is a lack of experimental evidence available in this area, partly due to the methodological difficulties involved but partly due to behaviour therapists underestimating its importance. Rosenthal (1966), in a series of studies, has drawn attention to the covert communication that occurs between the experimenter and subject in an experimental situation and demonstrated how this influences the subject's behaviour in the situation. In one experiment, the experimenter's expectations appeared to be responsible for about 50 per cent of the bias. It seems certain that similar influences, often covert, will occur within a therapeutic relationship. The therapist's expectation of treatment outcome correlates with actual outcome, and his prognostic assessment is influenced by the degree of congruence between his patient and himself in respect of socioeconomic background, educational level and personality traits. In a series of investigations of psychotherapy (mainly Rogerian), Truax and Carkhuff (1963, 1964; Truax, 1966a) have been able to demonstrate a positive correlation between the three therapist relationship variables of empathy, warmth and genuineness with successful therapeutic outcome. This work is impressive because it employed reliable rating scales of the relationship variables and it was possible to cross-validate the findings in a study of non-Rogerian psychotherapy. More recently, Truax *et al.* (1968) have reported that improvement in psychotherapy is also correlated with 'therapist potency' as rated by independent assessors. As described in chapter 1, Carl Rogers has emphasized that the three important factors he employs are largely attitudinal in nature and are not contingent upon specific verbalizations or behaviour of the patient. However, Truax (1966b) conducted another investigation which throws doubt on this. Five clinical psychologists rated randomly-selected samples of recordings of therapy sessions of a single successful case conducted by Rogers. Their findings indicated that he responded differentially to five of the nine aspects of the patient's behaviour studied, and significant increases in four out of the five classes of behaviour occurred. The therapist was more empathic and genuine when the patient made lucid statements, gave evidence of insight or expressed himself in a style similar to the therapist, so that a significant reinforcement effect could occur. This study demonstrates, above all, that a behavioural analysis can be made of some of the parameters involved in psychotherapy. Truax pointed out that one could profitably investigate the effect of rate, intensity and schedules of reinforcement on the specific behaviours selected for reinforcement. These findings, as well as the work on verbal conditioning and covert communication, show that the therapist can influence the patient unwittingly in non-directive therapy, so that one must bear this in mind when assessing the validity of psychodynamic theory from therapeutic material.

There is similar evidence that therapist and relationship variables influence the outcome of behaviour therapy. Schmidt *et al.* (1965), for example, compared the results of behaviour therapy carried out by four psychologists who had similar backgrounds and theoretical orientation. Inter-therapist comparisons revealed significant differences in the number of patients who improved with treatment and the number who terminated treatment prematurely. Koenig and Masters (1965) attempted to assess three types of treatment (desensitization, aversion and supportive counselling) with habitual smokers. Seven therapists each treated two subjects with the three treatment methods for nine sessions. Amount of reduction in smoking was unrelated to the particular method of treatment given but was significantly related to therapists. Successful treatment was correlated positively with the patients' expectation of outcome and negatively with their rating of positive qualities in their therapist. But this cannot be considered a crucial test of the efficacy of treatment techniques in smoking because it is unlikely that a single method of treatment would be expected to induce therapeutic change. Crisp (1966) found some evidence of a relationship between clinical change during behaviour therapy and the patient's attitude towards the therapist measured by a repertory grid technique.

Many therapists consider that a permissive attitude is an important condition for therapeutic change. It is argued that the permissive acceptance by the therapist of his patient's anxiety-arousing feelings and thoughts will lead to the reduction of anxiety. Partial experimental support for this is provided by Ditties (1957a and 1957b) who showed that a gradual decrease in the patient's anxiety (as measured by GSR) and avoidance behaviour occurred when the therapist adopted a permissive attitude.

Clearly it is possible to identify and measure some of the processes involved in therapeutic relationships which contribute to behaviour change. Theoretical formulations of these processes and their importance obviously differ. Role theory, transference or learning principles appear to differ in the language and concepts used but are describing similar processes. It is possible, for instance, to account for the emotional relationship that develops between patient and therapist in terms of psychoanalytic transference to the therapist of emotional feelings experienced in childhood towards parents or in terms of classical conditioning in which the therapist is a CS evoking emotional reactions, or in terms of operant conditioning with the therapist acting as a powerful source of discriminative and reinforcing stimuli, particularly social ones. Bandura has continuously emphasized how the psychotherapist may act as an esteemed model whose attitudes, values and patterns of behaviour will be imitated by the patient. If the patient is rewarded by the therapist in any way, the therapist's opinions acquire secondary reinforcement value.

Some of the investigations of behaviour therapy described in this book have attempted to control for 'non-specific' variables such as the therapeutic relationship and its duration. There is impressive evidence, for instance, in the studies of Davison, Gelder and Paul, that improvement in some fears and phobic disorders cannot be accounted for solely in terms of these, but that there is some extra factor in systematic desensitization which is responsible for better outcome. Nevertheless, it is extremely difficult to control effectively for 'non-specific' factors when the demand situation, therapist and patient expectancies and type of therapeutic relationship may be covertly and uniquely associated with a particular treatment technique. For this reason, it must be borne in mind that all the investigations of treatment which attempt to control for 'therapeutic relationship' are only able to control for a specific type of relationship (which the results show is often not 'therapeutic'). Discussion of neutral topics or a forty-five-minute interview discussing the possible origins of anxiety will establish a different relationship to the kind which develops when a therapist is engaged in a more active role in conducting systematic desensitization, implosive therapy, abreaction, suggestion, hypnotic, or non-directive therapy. The relationship is also influenced by personality variables and expectations of therapist and patient. It is, therefore, virtually impossible to control satisfactorily for 'relationship'. In other words, it seems impossible to isolate relationship from the type of transaction which is taking place. Because of these considerations, control for relationship must inevitably remain relatively crude. It is a justifiable criticism that behaviour therapists began by paying too little attention to these variables. Discovery of the relevant factors and processes involved and their systematic employment in treatment will no doubt increase the over-all efficacy of therapy. It is probable that relationship variables play a relatively greater role in some types of treatment and with some types of patient than in others. In patients with interpersonal anxiety, and in treatments employing operant conditioning or modelling, the therapeutic relationship may play a larger role than it does in the desensitization of a patient with a monosymptomatic phobia. Donner and Guerney (1969) have shown that desensitization of volunteers with test anxiety was almost as effective when administered by automated tape as when given by a therapist. The kind of relationship required may differ according to the method of treatment and type of patient. A permissive therapeutic atmosphere may be helpful for patients with an excess of anxiety and guilt whereas it might hamper the discriminative learning to be acquired by a patient with antisocial conduct.

There has been considerable discussion in the literature concerning the importance of the patients' motivation, anxiety level and personality type in prognosis. Limited, and sometimes contradictory research findings are available. The most consistent finding is that subjects with more widespread anxiety or neurotic symptoms respond less well to behaviour therapy. This could be explained in terms of a theory which holds that anxiety acts as an indiscriminate drive in the habits it energizes (generality of motivation – Kimble, 1961). Thus the presence of anxiety from any source, external or internal, may hamper attempts to treat any individual symptom alone. At present, however, generalized anxiety is not an absolute contra-indication to behaviour therapy, but is likely to require a combination of treatment methods. Motivation must always be of importance in bringing a patient to treatment and maintaining his co-operation, and is likely to influence its outcome.

In summary, research in this area is beginning to establish systematically the effect of such intangibles as the therapeutic relationship and expectations which the clinician has already been aware of intuitively if not in a form which allowed them to be experimentally manipulated or led to testable hypotheses. The stage is now being reached in which it is possible to restate these processes in terms of learning principles and general psychology. Behaviour therapy should not disregard these aspects of therapy but should utilize them within their theoretical framework. The non-specific factors discussed in this chapter enter inevitably into any form of treatment and it is naïve to consider that any therapeutic procedure can be administered in its pristine form.

In our view, behaviour therapy is a therapeutic approach based on the explicit and systematic application of learning principles derived from experimental psychological or clinical findings. It does not stem from any specific theory of psychology nor does it necessarily offer standardized treatments for specific disorders. No therapeutic strategy is excluded, provided that it is designed for the maximum exploitation of learning processes.

Chapter 8

Clinical Application of Behavior Therapy

In this chapter we discuss some of the problems which confront the behaviour therapist working in a clinical setting in the treatment of psychiatric disorder. Problems arise in the selection of patients, selection of symptoms to be treated, method of treatment, selection of therapist, and in the conduct of treatment. An attempt is made to discuss these topics in a constructive manner based on our experience with a variety of behaviour therapy methods employed in the treatment of 150 patients, the majority of whom were suffering from psychoneurotic disorders with a preponderance of phobic anxiety states.

As a result of behaviour therapy's link with experimental psychology, the majority of behaviour therapists are psychologists who are not medically qualified. They are therefore not qualified to carry out a medical assessment and treatment of patients who may have physical disease or require medical treatment. In addition, medical procedures such as drugs for relaxation or pharmacological aversion are employed in some behaviour therapy techniques. Apart from these considerations, treatment of patients, in Great Britain, takes place within the framework of a professional setting in which the patient and therapist have recognized roles and both may have some confidence because of well-established professional rules of conduct backed by legal sanctions. Because of this it is customary (and usually in the interest of patients and protection of non-medical personnel involved in their treatment) for a psychiatrist to be responsible for the over-all management of any patient. He will undertake the initial diagnostic assessment of new patients and may then refer those whom he considers might benefit from behaviour therapy to a suitable therapist. If the therapist agrees that behaviour therapy is indicated, he will carry out the treatment, but will share therapeutic responsibility with the psychiatrist. For obvious reasons, therefore, the psychiatrist will be cautious about the referral of patients and will be anxious to know the behaviour therapist's diagnostic formulation about each patient and the exact therapeutic procedure he proposes to adopt. The psychiatrist's anxiety may be enhanced by particular treatment techniques which involve exposure of the patient and therapist to procedures such as aversion therapy or practical retraining which fall outside the scope of traditionally accepted professional medical treatment. Sometimes the psychiatrist may restrict these procedures to safeguard his professional interests and reputation. In general it is probably in the ultimate interests of patients that dual responsibility exists. It is clearly going to work most satisfactorily when there is good communication and understanding between psychologist and psychiatrist. Unfortunately this happy state of affairs does not always exist. The situation is aggravated by some writers on behaviour therapy who make arrogant attacks on other approaches to mental disorders and make exaggerated claims for its therapeutic efficacy and its basis in 'modern learning theory'. This gives the impression that the behaviour therapist has at his disposal a panacea consisting of a repertoire of well-established, routine methods of treatment. As we have seen this is far from true and such an erroneous presentation leads to false expectancies and over-optimism or aversion to behavioural methods.

Such controversy, although useful in having stimulated rethinking about theory and experimental and clinical investigation, is generally agreed to have shed more heat than light. Careful discussion between behaviour therapists, psychotherapists and psychiatrists leads to the learning of each other's language and to better understanding. In our own experience it usually also leads to the discovery of large areas of agreement in aetiological assessment and possible lines of treatment. No one has a monopoly of truth and all methods of treatment achieve some success.

Selection of patients for behaviour therapy

At the present time the psychiatrist, assuming he is prepared to consider behaviour therapy, is most likely to refer patients whose psychiatric disorder can be conceptualized most easily as an s–r paradigm. In practice, patients with relatively isolated phobias or behaviour anomalies form the bulk of referrals. Patients with more widespread symptoms such as generalized anxiety, depersonalization and compulsive symptoms, and evidence of poor adjustment in most areas of life (akin to the diagnostic categories of mixed neurosis and personality disorders), are much less likely to be referred, as are patients with psychoses. These selection criteria have been strengthened by the early published reports that behaviour therapy is most successful with isolated specific symptoms. Another type of referral, increasingly common in our department, is of patients who have presented depression or complex neurotic disorders which have improved with drug treatment or psychotherapy but who are left with some specific symptoms such as phobias or compulsive rituals which could be amenable to behaviour therapy. A third type of referral consists of complex disorders which have not responded to other therapeutic methods and behaviour treatment is considered as a final resort.

From a pragmatic viewpoint, these selection criteria are understandable in our present state of knowledge and serve as rough guides. However, in the light of growing evidence that behaviour therapy techniques can be successfully employed in some of the complex neuroses and psychoses, these selection criteria will need to be modified. In fact our own data suggest that there is no close relationship between classification of disorders into 'simple' and 'complex' and their response to behaviour therapy. Some patients with monosymptomatic phobias did not improve, whereas some with longstanding and extensive disorders, referred as a last resort, improved to a surprising degree. The problem is that there are few established criteria for predicting response to behaviour therapy and there are no absolute contra-indications.

At the initial diagnostic assessment it is useful to make a formal psychiatric diagnosis. This often indicates the first choice of treatment, such as physical treatments in the majority of organic and functional psychoses. In the less clearly defined neurotic and behaviour disturbances it is important to determine whether they are associated with a psychotic disorder or are the consequence of treatable physical illness, in which case behaviour therapy is unlikely to be the first line of treatment. However, the majority of neurotic and behaviour disorders are not associated with psychosis or resultant on treatable physical illness. We have seen how complex the factors responsible for initiating and maintaining disordered behaviour can be. A detailed psychiatric history and phenomenological analysis of the symptoms are required as well as a detailed behavioural analysis. A psychodynamic formulation may be of practical assistance to the behaviour therapist as well as to the psychiatrist. There is almost unanimous agreement among experienced behaviour therapists that their most difficult task is the initial analysis of the patient's symptoms upon which a rational treatment programme depends. This involves the identification of the most relevant problems of the patient and the dimensions along which therapy should proceed. Simply asking a patient what his main problem is or just observing his behaviour is not sufficient. Such a restricted and naïve approach often leads to an inadequate analysis and misapplication of therapy. A few examples will illustrate this. Repeated examination failure in a University student could be due to one or more of several factors such as insufficient intelligence, abnormal slowness of mental functioning, a high anxiety level, depression, obsessional checking and rechecking the accuracy of his responses, intrusion of irrelevant thoughts, or insufficient or inefficient preparation for the exams. Several of these factors may be operating together and obviously different methods of treatment may be required according to the main determinants of the academic failure. A child may present an apparently isolated symptom of school refusal. This could be due to anxiety evoked by some aspect of the school situation, anxiety due to separation from home, or the availability of more rewarding pastimes such as being indulged by mother, visiting the funfair or stealing from gas-meters. Here again, more than one factor may be operating and suitable treatment will depend on accurate diagnosis. Counterconditioning may be required for anxiety when its source is identified, operant conditioning involving parents and schoolteachers may lead to appropriate modification of reinforcements so that attending school becomes more rewarding. Agoraphobia, claustrophobia, and social phobias are commonly found to be complex disorders and identification of the anxiety-evoking cues and their dimensions can be very difficult to assess. Agoraphobia may

216

arise largely as the result of a previous frightening experience in the street such as a road accident, or apprehension at the possibility of meeting strangers or friends in the case of interpersonal anxiety. Agoraphobia may be reinforced by a relative who may be gratified by the patient's dependency on him. Often the agoraphobic is aware of specific conflicts or fears in a particular phobic situation, for example a fear of dying or an obsessional fear of killing someone or a wish to exhibit themselves. Secondary gains such as gratification for being treated as an invalid or not having to go to work may play a significant role in maintaining the symptoms. Phobias may result from the absence of appropriate responses due to lack of suitable learning rather than the disruptive effect of anxiety. Lack of social skills or of the ability to be appropriately assertive may be the underlying basis of situational phobias.

It is always important to establish whether anxiety is responsible for the maintenance of individual symptoms. For instance, encopresis is sometimes due to the pleasure of self-soiling or reinforcement by a concerned mother rather than to fear of using the lavatory or of painful defecation. Motor disorders such as compulsive rituals may or may not be mediated by anxiety. Direct modification of the instrumental response may be required. Similarly, in psychotic patients, it would be a mistake to assume that the disordered behaviour is always the result of unsuitable schedules of environmental reinforcement. Some symptoms may be mediated by anxiety or by cognitive processes and treatment directed to these would be more suitable.

Behavioural analysis becomes more difficult the more complex the case is. Sometimes the initial impression may be that a variety of symptoms can be subsumed under one heading. A patient may complain of a fear of travelling on trains or buses, going to cinemas and theatres, attending official meetings or parties, and of sexual relationships. These different phobias might all be subsumed under the dimension of confinement with people. But it would still be necessary to determine the specific sources of anxiety in each of these situations. The patient may have previously had fainting attacks in such a situation, or been severely criticized, or experienced frightening aggressive impulses towards other people. A fear of rejection or failure may be the basis of multiple phobias. In this case one might attempt to desensitize the fear of failure in social activities rather than treat each situational phobia separately.

Another type of problem is encountered with patients who have a number of apparently unrelated symptoms at the level of behavioural analysis. A patient may present with anorexia nervosa but also drink heavily and complain of agoraphobia and depersonalization. Another patient's main complaint was inability to cope with his job, but in addition displayed compulsive hand-washing, timidity and submissiveness with people in authority, impotence with his wife, and episodes of depression. One could try to treat all the symptoms concurrently, or select the symptom considered to be the most basic. Unfortunately the therapist often has no certain means of evaluating whether symptoms are independent or dependent on a 'fundamental' disorder and therefore has difficulty in planning treatment. He may be guided initially in these cases by a psychodynamic formulation which structures the multiplicity of symptoms. Empirical evaluation of different methods of selecting the symptoms to be treated is required.

Recently several attempts have been made to construct rating scales (Fear Survey Schedules) which will provide a measure of the range and intensity of specific fears and a total score of 'fearfulness' (Wolpe and Lang, 1964; Geer, 1965; Manosevitz and Lanyon, 1965). Some research has been carried out to determine their reliability and validity (e.g. Grossberg and Wilson, 1965; Lanyon and Manosevitz, 1966; Cooke, 1966; Rubin et al., 1968). These scales have been offered to research workers and clinicians for designing treatment and assessing changes. They appear to be reliable and valid in so far as they tend to be related to measures of observable behaviour in fear-evoking situations. But Rubin et al. (1968), in a factor analysis of a fifty-one-item fear inventory, found that the items were drawn from four major areas and were not entirely independent fears. It might therefore be misleading to use the total score as a means of selecting samples of subjects for comparative studies. Another important point is that the fear schedules have been validated on non-psychiatric populations and their relevance to psychiatric patients remains to be established. General inventories of anxiety such as the Taylor Manifest Anxiety Scale (Taylor, 1953) have a very limited usefulness in this context because they do not identify specific fears. In addition all questionnaires can be faked or influenced by response styles. Some indirect methods such as measures of autonomic reactivity overcome some of the disadvantages of questionnaires, but they do not always correlate with the subjective experience of anxiety and the presence of clinical symptoms. At present, therefore, as already discussed, they are more useful as research tools than as practical aids to designing treatment.

The manner in which the patient conceptualizes the world including his experiences and symptoms may well prove to be a more relevant guide to the analysis of his behaviour disorder. If this proves to be the case, Kelly's Repertory Grid Technique (Kelly, 1955), in which a systematic study of the meaning and the relationships between the concepts employed by an individual patient in structuring his personal experiences can be carried out, may become a useful means of tracing the relationships of specific symptoms to each other. At present, however, careful clinical examination, supplemented by information obtained from other informants and direct observation of behaviour, remain the best method of assessment. The therapist is obliged to adopt a pragmatic approach and select for treatment the symptoms which appear the most incapacitating and 'central' and which may be amenable to available behavioural methods. If the response to the initial plan of treatment is poor, reappraisal of the patient's disturbance in the light of any further information gleaned during treatment will be required. Clearly, when presented with a number of symptoms, there is a choice either of selecting one or a few symptoms for initial treatment, or attempting to treat all symptoms simultaneously. Lazarus suggests that complex disorders require a barrage of methods directed against modifying all the symptoms right from the start (Lazarus, 1966b; Lazarus and Serber, 1968). However, this can lead to unnecessary therapeutic activity as well as presenting practical difficulties in its execution, because improvement of a treated symptom often leads to improvement in others not receiving specific attention. Improvement in agoraphobia could lead to improved occupational adjustment, financial status, less social isolation and relief of anxiety and depression. The difficulty lies in predicting in advance 'key symptoms' whose amelioration will be associated with more widespread improvement. Developmental history, behavioural analysis, and psychodynamic formulations may sometimes successfully identify such symptoms. Wilson and Evans (1967), have attempted to explain the occurence of widespread improvement following the treatment of a specific symptom in terms of the Hullian concept of behaviour consisting of a series of different habit-family hierarchies. If one hierarchy is reinforced or extinguished, other members of the same family tend to be affected similarly. Unfortunately this hypothesis does not help to determine precisely in advance how many family hierarchies are involved in a patient's behaviour anomalies. Its lack of predictive value makes it more of a *post hoc* explanation.

Behaviour therapy has been widely criticized not only for its theoretical assumptions regarding aetiology which are considered too naïve and trivial, but also for its therapeutic practices which imply manipulation and control of the patient's behaviour. We have argued that such criticisms are not justified. While we would emphasize the fundamental importance of an humanitarian approach and respect for the individual, the aesthetic satisfaction of sophisticated philosophy should not take precedence over other theoretical models which have been shown empirically to be more effective in helping the patient. Patients who place a high value on self-understanding and insight may be at a disadvantage if they suffer from psychiatric disorders which respond less well to 'insight psychotherapy' than to behaviour therapy, because they will be much less motivated towards the latter type of treatment. Obviously the patient's own attitudes and expectations must be taken into account if only because of their potential influence in determining the outcome of treatment. When diagnostic assessment has appraised the relative importance of cognitive, affective and behavioural factors in a particular disorder and a particular behaviour therapy technique appears to be the treatment of choice, an explanation of its rationale should be given.

. Usually the therapist also presents experimental and clinical evidence demonstrating the efficacy of the method. There is much to recommend this practice, which serves to structure the therapeutic situation and mobilize expectancy and suggestion towards a satisfactory outcome. The therapist, as opposed to the research investigator, should try to make maximal use of therapeutic aids. Naturally there are dangers attached to over-enthusiastic or misleading approaches. In our view, a realistic explanation with emphasis on the importance of the patient's active participation and co-operation should be adopted.

When a particular symptom has been selected for treatment, difficulty may be encountered in bringing it under experimental control. For example, if phobic anxiety is to be treated by desensitization, it is important that the patient does not experience anxiety through exposure to phobic cues outside the treatment situation. An isolated phobia of snakes would not present a problem because they can be avoided fairly easily. But an agoraphobic with extensive fears and frequent panic attacks may have great difficulty in avoiding anxiety-evoking situations outside of treatment. Many such patients need to be admitted to hospital on account of this, but even then it may prove very difficult to provide an anxiety-free environment. Symptoms such as obsessional thoughts and rituals, motor tics and stammering are often very difficult to prevent outside the treatment situation. Considerable ingenuity may be required to bring them under any sort of stimulus control, and hospitalization with continuous supervision and some restriction of activity may be required.

Choice of method of treatment

With many symptoms there is a choice of more than one behavioural technique. Psychogenic vomiting or compulsive rituals could be treated by systematic desensitization, flooding, aversion therapy, positive conditioning, operant conditioning, or a combination of methods. The point to be made is that there is no standardized or rigid application of particular methods for particular symptoms. The planning of treatment involves a flexible approach to the individual patient with a careful assessment of aetiology. If the symptom is currently mediated by anxiety, desensitization may be the initial treatment choice. If it is considered to be maintained by secondary gains (increased attention for example) operant conditioning may be the first choice. If anxiety is no longer maintaining an instrumental response, aversion therapy or negative practice may be appropriate. When the symptom is thought to be due to the absence of some class of behaviour responses (for example, lack of social skills), training by instruction, imitation and shaping may be undertaken first. Sometimes there may be difficulty in deciding whether to treat the husband or wife, parent or child. The choice may lie between trying to modify the hostility of one or the passivity of the other. Obviously it is often appropriate to treat both, either together or separately. In deciding on the method of treatment to be employed, the therapist must be guided by his diagnostic assessment and knowledge of suitable techniques. Often the plan of treatment is modified according to the progress of the patient and in the light of further knowledge of the variables influencing his behaviour. Furthermore, there is some experimental evidence that personality variables may be of relevance in the choice of treatment. For instance, Eysenck (1968b) has suggested that the effects of punishment are influenced by the dimension of extraversion. Praise is a more effective reinforcer in introverts, punishment in extroverts. More research is required, however, before they can be accurately applied in the individual patient.

Problems associated with treatment techniques

The administration of treatment is often beset with difficulties. In part this is because there are no standard administration procedures. Opinions differ on 'crucial procedural factors' and their violation is not always demonstrably detrimental. Most difficulties arise because of individual differences in patients' responses to particular procedures.

In systematic desensitization there may be great difficulty in constructing the anxiety hierarchies. Apart from the problem already discussed of whether the symptoms can be considered under one single theme, there may be difficulty in identifying the variables which influence the intensity of anxiety evoked. The patient often does not know the particular cues which generate anxiety and he has to be carefully questioned and asked to imagine or be placed in particular situations so that his response can be observed. He may have avoided the phobic situation for years and have little memory or even experience of it. Distance, size and activity are often important in animal phobias. But in two patients who did not respond to systematic desensitization in imagination it emerged during practical retraining that sudden and unexpected movement of the animal was the main factor leading to anxiety and this had not been included in the original anxiety hierarchies.

There is no accurate method of constructing the hierarchy items so that each item represents an equal increase in anxiety. Fortunately this is probably not necessary. The patient is asked to rank each item himself, and this may be supplemented by ranking real life situations. If difficulty is encountered in desensitization of the next item, intermediate items can be introduced in an *ad hoc* manner. Occasionally, rearrangement of the hierarchy may be required. When the reliability of the ranking is in doubt, the item cards should be shuffled so that the patient can grade the hierarchy again and discrepancies can be resolved.

In counterconditioning procedures, muscle relaxation has been employed most frequently as the incompatible response. In some patients, muscular relaxation is difficult to attain, or if attained is not accompanied by subjective feelings of calm and relaxation. Muscular relaxation is often unsuccessful in children. Some patients appear to have specific fears concerning relaxation and hypnosis which they express in terms of a fear of losing control or of making an exhibition of themselves or a fear of being dominated by the therapist. At times these fears can be circumvented by modification of technique and emphasis placed on the patient retaining active control of himself. It may be possible to desensitize the patient's anxiety regarding relaxation. Alternative methods described in chapter 4, such as emotive imagery or anxiety-relief, could be used if muscular relaxation cannot be used, but experience of these methods is limited and their efficiency is not yet well established.

Another alternative to instruction in muscle relaxation is the use of drugs such as diazepam or methohexitone sodium. Here again there is less clinical experience of this method and theoretical and practical problems arise. A theoretical difficulty is that sedative drugs might impede conditioning. Practical difficulties are encountered in patients who have a dislike or fear of injections or medications, or when the medication leads to unpleasant mood disturbances or abreaction, or if drug dependence develops (Reed, 1966; Sergeant and Yorkston, 1968). Some preliminary reports of the use of drug-induced relaxation have been encouraging and further investigation is warranted (Brady, 1966, 1967; Friedman, 1966a; Friedman and Silverstone, 1967; Kraft, 1967; Worsley and Freeman, 1967). The poor results obtained by Yorkston *et al.* (1968) have been discussed in chapter 6. On the basis

of Davison's theory of the importance of self-induced muscle relaxation and a consideration of the influence of cognitive factors, Davison
and Valins (1968) suggested that, when drugs are used for relaxation,
it should be emphasized to the patient that the drug is merely helping
him to relax himself and his relaxation is not purely drug induced. It
would appear that Brady uses this technique when employing methohexitone. Davison and Valins comment that the efficacy of tranquillizer
drugs in general may be improved by stressing to the patient that he
is relaxing himself and encouraging him to appreciate that he is no
longer anxious in situations which previously evoked anxiety.

Difficulties can arise in achieving a graduated exposure to the
hierarchy items if the patient finds it difficult or impossible to imagine
them, or experiences no anxiety when imagining them. An attempt can
be made to get the patient to use all sense modalities when constructing
the image, because often subjects are more proficient in some modalities than others. The patient can be asked to describe the items aloud
(Badri, 1967), or pictures or tape recordings may be used if they are
found to elicit anxiety.

Duration of exposure to each item is timed from the onset of a clear
image. The therapist is therefore dependent on the patient signalling
to him when he is imagining a scene or experiencing anxiety. It is usual
for the therapist to take note also of any overt behaviour such as movement or facial expression which may be manifestations of anxiety even
in the absence of the patient signalling. 'Anxiety' has experiential,
behavioural and autonomic components and it would be unwise to
ignore any of its manifestations. Lazarus (1968d) recommends that the
patient be questioned after every scene presentation to check that he
is imagining the scene effectively and to determine his emotional state.
Despite careful monitoring of desensitization therapy, some patients
relapse in the sense that they exhibit anxiety to items already successfully desensitized. Sometimes this seems to be the result of a panic
attack or exposure to a phobic situation not yet desensitized occurring
before the next treatment session. Whatever the reason for relapse, it
is necessary to inquire for this at the start of each session and to repeat
desensitization if necessary.

Desensitization in imagination may be successfully completed
without any therapeutic gain if no generalization to real life situations

has taken place. In our own experience this occurs more frequently when the phobic stimulus (e.g. flying, thunderstorms) is one which commonly evokes mild anxiety in many people. When generalization to real life stimuli does not occur, an attempt should be made to use more lifelike stimuli with the aid of photographs and recordings, or, when feasible, practical retraining. The greater efficacy of the latter has been demonstrated in snake phobic volunteers by Barlow *et al.* (1969). Obvious difficulties arise in arranging graded stimuli in real life for certain phobias such as thunderstorms, agoraphobia and many social phobias. In addition such procedures are time-consuming for the therapist and there may be difficulty in maintaining a suitable counter-conditioning response in real life so that anxiety is not experienced.

Because of these considerations, a treatment approach which combines desensitization in imagination with practical retraining may prove to be of value. When the phobic stimulus is one which can be brought into the consulting room, successful desensitization to an imagined stimulus is followed immediately by presentation of the real stimulus while the patient is relaxed and then in his normal state. When the phobic stimulus cannot be introduced into the treatment room, for example with an agoraphobic, the patient is made familiar with a particular journey while accompanied by the therapist. The journey is then divided into graduated stages of increasing distance. He is desensitized in imagination to travelling the shortest distance and is then required to actually make the trip. In between treatment sessions he is encouraged to practise the items already desensitized, and to repeat desensitization in imagination before starting the journey if he doubts his ability to achieve it without anxiety. This approach combines some of the advantages of both techniques and initial imaginal desensitization is likely to make the difficult fine grading of items in real life less necessary. Moreover, patients find the treatment procedure more realistic and appear to have more confidence in its efficiency. Concurrent practical retraining also allows a continuous assessment of progress and a degree of generalization to be made by the patient and therapist. Our preliminary results of a comparative investigation of desensitization in imagination and combined imaginal and *in vivo* treatment confirm the findings of Garfield *et al.* (1967) that combined treatment is superior.

The series of investigations reported by Bandura and his colleagues (Bandura, 1968) already referred to in previous chapters lends support to the hypothesis that the more realistic the phobic stimuli employed in treatment, the better the outcome in terms of elimination of avoidance responses. In this respect a combination of observation of a number of fearless live models combined with gradual participation by 'phobic' subjects in approach responses was more effective than mere observation of a live model alone. This in turn was more effective than observation of a symbolic model (cine film) or systematic desensitization in imagination (Bandura and Menlove, 1968; Ritter, 1968). It must be remembered that these results were obtained with subjects (including children) with specific animal 'phobias' and the findings require confirmation in psychiatric patients. However, they do suggest how modelling procedures and participation can be employed in combination with imaginal desensitization and practical retraining.

Aversion therapy raises certain ethical issues as well as theoretical and technical difficulties. Doctors and therapists must be concerned that they do not inflict more harm than good, and always have to decide when to treat rather than leave alone, and often have to choose between a variety of methods of varying efficacy and danger. This can lead to difficult clinical decisions in a wide variety of illnesses. The particular difficulties associated with aversion therapy are, firstly, the ethical and emotional attitudes concerning the use of punishment, and secondly, the types of behaviour disorder for which aversion therapy is used. Although punishment is often sanctioned by Government and employed by parents and teachers, a large number of people, including doctors, have an abhorrence or strong reluctance of using punishment as a method of treating patients. If, however, it is the most effective or the only treatment available for a disorder which will cause worse suffering if left untreated, many doctors would agree to give and many patients would agree to receive aversion therapy. The second difficulty mentioned arises because many of the disorders for which aversion therapy might be the most effective treatment arouse more social disapproval and suffering to society than to the individual himself. Alcoholism and sexual deviations often come into this category. Here again careful consideration must be given to the individual case. An alcoholic with cirrhosis of the liver who asks for treatment to help him stop drinking is not likely to be refused treatment because it is unjustified on moral grounds. If aversion therapy appeared to be the most likely treatment to succeed, or other methods had already been unsuccessful, many doctors might be prepared to undertake it. Similarly a patient seeking treatment for transvestism accompanied by anxiety, guilt and depression with suicidal wishes, whose family life and work are adversely affected, should not have psychiatric advice withheld. Psychiatric assessment may point to a number of lines of approach such as symptomatic treatment of his anxiety and depression with drugs, or an attempt to relieve anxiety and guilt and allow the patient to accept his transvestism by desensitization or psychotherapy, an attempt to modify hostile and intolerant feelings of his wife or family to his cross-dressing or an attempt to modify or eliminate his transvestism by means of insight psychotherapy or aversion therapy. The choice of treatment method in this case should be based on clinical considerations of the likely beneficial effects balanced against the risks. If aversion therapy was selected on this basis, many doctors might feel it was justifiable. Fortunately, there is not often much difficulty in deciding whether or not aversion therapy is ethically justifiable for a particular patient. It goes without saying that the nature of the treatment must be explained to the patient and he must give his consent. The quality of the consent must be taken into account, particularly if the patient is being influenced strongly by someone else such as the Courts, a prison governor, employer or family. The psychiatrist may have more difficulty in deciding whether aversion therapy or indeed any psychiatric treatment is justified if the patient is referred primarily at the instigation of someone other than the patient, and he is not convinced that the patient is himself suffering as a result of his deviant behaviour and wants help in modifying it. In such cases there may well be genuine differences of opinion as to whether psychiatric treatment, particularly aversion therapy, is justified.

Problems are encountered in aversion therapy because of the uncertain effects of punishment which can sometimes lead to disruption of behaviour, increased anxiety and irritability, temporary suppression or even reinforcement of responses. It is not often possible to establish stable avoidance responses similar to those found in some 'naturally' occurring isolated phobias. As already discussed, when the behavioural response (e.g. alcohol addiction) is itself an instrumental response reducing anxiety, the establishment of an avoidance response to alcohol may leave the patient in a double-avoidance conflict in which he is worse off. These are probably the reasons responsible for some of the difficulties found in clinical practice. Depression, anxiety and hostility can arise during treatment, and lead to the patient refusing to continue with it. Periodic booster treatment may help to maintain the stability of the avoidance response but relapses are still too frequent. Probably the absence of more appropriate responses in the patient's behaviour contributes to this. A patient who is able to enjoy heterosexual intercourse is likely to find it easier to avoid engaging in homosexual behaviour than a patient whose only activity has been homosexual. The establishment of more adaptive responses can be a formidable task.

Difficulty can arise in finding a suitable aversive stimulus. Pharmacological aversion has several drawbacks already discussed. Habituation to electric shock can lead to difficulty and a few patients seem impervious to it. This does not seem to occur more frequently in masochistic patients because the stimuli which they find sexually arousing are usually highly specific ones. However, one must remain alert to the risk of inducing an electric shock fetishism with aversion therapy (Marks, 1968b).

The most common problems encountered in the treatment of enuresis by the bell and pad method are failure of the patient to be woken up by the alarm and difficulty in getting the patient to follow out the instructions correctly. Heavy sleeping may be counteracted by use of a louder alarm or stimulant drugs (e.g. methedrine) to lighten sleep. If patients are reluctant or unable to co-operate in the treatment, in-patient treatment may be required. In our experience, intermittent reinforcement and gradual removal of the apparatus and withdrawal of drugs (after initial arrest has been achieved) while in hospital and then at home has diminished the relapse rate.

The planning of operant conditioning techniques is often laborious and many difficulties are encountered in finding suitable rewards and subsequently arranging that consistent reinforcement schedules are received by the patient and that he is not exposed to different reinforcement contingencies outside the treatment situation which have no therapeutic effect. Many patients such as retarded depressives and withdrawn schizophrenics do not respond to social reinforcement and sometimes do not respond to primary or generalized rewards either. Where the response to be reinforced is not present in the patient's repertoire (e.g. speech in a mute schizophrenic), a very considerable amount of time may be required to establish it by imitation and shaping. Browning (1967) describes a procedure which allows the simultaneous comparison of the efficacy of different social reinforcement contingencies for a particular patient which may help the therapist to select the best reinforcement for treatment.

When an effective reinforcement has been found the next difficulty lies in ensuring that it is applied as consistently as possible by other people who come into contact with the patient. If he is in hospital it is important that the nursing staff co-operate in the operant conditioning programme. Professional staff have been trained to respond with sympathy and attention when their patients exhibit disturbed behaviour. This may have the effect of reinforcing the maladaptive behaviour which the therapist is trying to eliminate. Hospital patients tend to be better 'behaviour therapists' in so far as they more often ignore disordered behaviour of other patients than reward it. Their frequency of inappropriate reward was only 12 per cent (Gelfand *et al.*, 1967). On the other hand Buehler *et al.* (1966) in an investigation of social reinforcement in a corrective institution found that 70–80 per cent of the inmates' delinquent behaviour received social approval by other delinquents. Delinquent behaviour was significantly more frequently reinforced than punished, while socially conforming behaviour was more frequently punished than rewarded. Reinforcement by the staff tended to be inconsistent; this might be one reason for the generally accepted finding that delinquency may become more severe after institutionalization.

These studies strongly support clinical impressions and indicate the need for close co-operation between all members of staff and detailed exploration of the rationale and plan of treatment. Some staff are naturally reluctant to adopt a therapeutic role which may be at variance with their own concept of their role. They may be suspicious initially and their full co-operation may not be obtained until they witness the efficacy of such treatment and are satisfied that they are helping their patients.

There is often a disappointing lack of generalization of operant conditioning to life outside the hospital. A search must be made for inappropriate reinforcement contingencies being supplied by relatives or others in the patient's social environment which may be maintaining his symptoms. It may be possible to modify this and to treat the patient in the community. There is already a precedent for including members of the patient's family in the psychiatric treatment or larger groups still in therapeutic communities. When marital couples or other family members are included in treatment it may be necessary only to instruct the partner how to behave towards the 'patient' or the partner may himself require more active help to enable him to modify his own responses to the 'patient'. Most therapists find that it is helpful to see both husband and wife in cases of marital and sexual problems. They may be seen and treated separately but behaviour therapists as well as many psychotherapists suggest that combined treatment is more effective (Meyer and Crisp, 1966; Madsen and Ullmann, 1967; Lazarus, 1968c). Sometimes the marital partner can take an active part in the behaviour treatment of the patient's sexual difficulties.

General problems encountered in treatment

Apart from the problems associated with particular treatment methods, there are some difficulties encountered during behaviour therapy which are not peculiar to it alone, but occur also during other forms of psychiatric and medical treatment. Accurate assessment of the symptom under treatment, particularly repetitive motor symptoms, is essential if slight improvement is to be detected and premature termination or alteration of treatment avoided.

The motivation of the patient may fluctuate or diminish to the extent that he no longer co-operates in treatment or he may actively sabotage or terminate it. A relationship develops between the patient and behaviour therapist and both may become conscious or show evidence of strong positive or negative feelings towards each other. Hostility, admiration or dependency feelings can obviously have an effect on the progress of behaviour therapy, either enhancing or detrimental. Such relationship factors may be one cause of the fluctuations in mood and intensity of symptoms sometimes encountered during treatment. No practising behaviour therapist with clinical experience is likely not to have observed these phenomena in some patients. They appear to be identical with phenomena occurring during the course of psychoanalytical therapy and which are conceptualized in terms of transference and resistance. Sometimes changes in the clinical state of the patient seem related to current environmental factors such as extra stress at work or family illness. When changes in motivation or symptomatology do occur, the behaviour therapist must make a diagnostic appraisal of the new situation and further psychiatric assessment is indicated. Subsequent management will depend upon the factors thought to be responsible for the change. In any case it is important to look out for changes in the patient's life situation during behaviour therapy which may cause stress and impede his progress.

The psychiatric social worker may be able to help environmental factors, psychotropic drugs may be prescribed for sustained anxiety or depressive mood disturbance. If interaction in the therapeutic relationship is thought to be responsible for the change, a number of courses of action are possible. The view may be taken that interpersonal problems are of primary importance and require to be treated before, for example, proceeding with the systematic desensitization of a travel phobia. In other cases relationship factors may not seem to be of such prime importance and it may be decided to continue behaviour therapy for the symptom under treatment while, at the same time, trying to prevent strong emotional feelings towards the therapist from interfering. This may be attempted by allowing the patient to discuss his feelings and giving him some explanation and reassurance. Whether or not specific behavioural procedures are adopted or the therapist refers the patient for some other psychiatric treatment will depend on clinical reassessment.

Some clinicians consider that concurrent administration of psychotherapy and behaviour therapy is feasible (e.g. Marks and Gelder, 1966; Meyer and Crisp, 1966). Our own more recent experience has emphasized the difficulties that can arise in combined treatment. Close communication between psychotherapist and behaviour therapist is essential. There must be a clear understanding of the aims and methods of each and these must be explained to the patient. Particularly during the early stages of insight psychotherapy the presence of symptoms and some degree of anxiety and depression may act as an incentive to the patient to 'work' in treatment. Furthermore, analytical interpretations may increase his anxiety level. Behaviour therapy may interfere with psychotherapy by affording the patient a means of escape from analytic work. Psychotherapy may interfere with behaviour therapy if it leads to high anxiety levels which hinder systematic desensitization. Obviously the two forms of treatment cannot always be combined, particularly during the earlier stages of analytical psychotherapy. However, there are times when it might be advantageous to combine psychotherapy with behaviour therapy or to precede behaviour therapy with psychotherapy. In fact, some form of 'psychotherapy' in the sense of support, encouragement, explanation and guidance is often necessary and beneficial during behaviour therapy and can be conceptualized in terms of learning processes. Examples where concurrent insight psychotherapy and behaviour therapy are feasible are afforded by patients in psychotherapy who are making some generalized improvement but who have discrete symptoms such as an isolated phobia or alcohol dependence which might respond to systematic desensitization or aversion therapy.

Difficulties sometimes arise in terminating treatment and discharging patients from hospital. There may be anxiety or successfully treated symptoms may return. This is likely to be due to apprehension about functioning without symptoms in the less secure everyday environment and a reluctance to give up relationships associated with positive reward. Clearly this touches on similar aspects discussed in the preceding paragraphs. In order to anticipate difficulties over discharge of patients, efforts should be made to prevent overdependency developing during treatment by encouraging the patient to retain contact with his outside environment and relationships while in hospital and in arranging that he goes home for gradually increasing periods of time as he improves and the time for discharge approaches. The patient may start work from hospital or attend hospital as a day patient and sleep at home to ease the transition. In some cases it may be helpful for the patient to receive some behaviour therapy in his own environment.

There are no hard and fast rules concerning the frequency and duration of follow-up required. Relapses are most likely to occur at times when environmental stress may occur, such as the transition period from hospital to home and restarting work. Patients usually like to retain contact with the hospital and their therapist. They may obtain reassurance and support from out-patient interviews and frequent initial follow-up at weekly intervals is recommended. According to subsequent progress the frequency of visits is gradually diminished. Our own clinical practice is to follow up patients for at least a year. Patients treated with aversion therapy are the most likely to relapse, so that close observation and booster treatments are required.

We have only been able to discuss briefly in the short space available some of the most common problems encountered with behaviour therapy in clinical practice. Emphasis has been given to the difficulties that can arise, the limitations of treatment, and the demands made on the clinical judgement, intuition and ingenuity of those who carry out behaviour therapy to resolve the problems for which 'modern learning theory' does not provide set answers. Although their work is often routine or frustrating, many behaviour therapists find the problems challenging and exciting.

Chapter 9

Conclusion:
Behavior Therapy –
Present Status and Prospects

Present status

It has been said that behaviour therapy has reached the dangerous stage at which the initial enthusiasm and optimism which sustains any new cult or therapeutic method starts to falter as reports of its failures and limitations accumulate. The onset of disillusionment is followed by a catastrophic fall in success rate because its therapeutic efficacy is denuded of its powerful placebo effect. Physicians are familiar with the advice to use new remedies while they still have the power to heal. The next stage in the history of new therapies is a critical reappraisal which may result in a more sober assessment of their value and the discovery of resemblances to other existing forms of treatment. To some extent behaviour therapy has followed this path. It was oversold initially and subsequent investigations have shown that its value is not limitless. As difficulties have been encountered, its theoretical formulations and therapeutic procedures have tended to expand in an *ad hoc* manner. It is accused of being inhuman and ineffective, or human and effective only because of its rediscovery and employment of well-established psychotherapeutic procedures. It is criticized on the grounds that it does not derive from established learning theory because there is no established learning theory. Its use of the terms 'stimulus' and 'response' is considered plagiaristic because they bear such little resemblance to the physiologist's use of them, or degrading because it ignores every uniquely human aspect of man.

We have tried to present a balanced account of the theory and practice of behaviour therapy in the preceding chapters. There is some truth in many of the criticisms but, despite this, behaviour therapy has reached the stage at which it has established itself as a useful and promising approach to psychiatric disorder and an effective method of treatment for some conditions. With regard to its semantic and theoretical

framework, stimulus and response are best defined by their relationship to each other (see Hocutt, 1967; Kimble, 1967). Central processes
are recognized by all learning theorists; they differ in their choice of
intervening variables or theoretical constructs. As behaviour therapists
recognize the importance of interpersonal relationships and experiential meaning in the genesis and modification of psychiatric disorder
their theory and methods will come to have some resemblance to other
psychotherapeutic approaches. However, behaviour therapy is likely
to retain some identity of its own by its explicit attempt to employ
learning principles in its therapeutic methods. Accurate identification
of the factors upon which psychiatric symptoms are currently contingent, and their behavioural modification by counterconditioning or
the acquisition of more adaptive responses by shaping, imitation and
the establishment of generalized reinforcers, will be prominent
features of the behaviour therapy approach. Behaviourists have for
long been promising that they will turn their attention to thinking
processes and attempt to encompass these within a learning framework. Clinical experience with behaviour therapy has served as an
impetus in this direction.

Early behaviourist formulations were characterized by a rigidly
narrow concentration on overt behaviour and a doctrinaire disregard
of physiological, biochemical and experiential processes. While there
is some advantage in exploring to its limits the explanatory and predictive power of a 'pure' behavioural approach, its successful integration with other methods of approach must inevitably lead to
greater knowledge and be of pragmatic value to the therapist. Because
of the intentionally restricted approach of early behaviourism, it was
only natural that behaviour therapy was initially employed for relatively discrete and isolated disorders. In justification of this, behaviour
therapy has been found to be more effective in these disorders in
'normal' subjects than in the more widespread disorders found in
many psychiatric patients. Although we do not think that it has quite
reached the stage of providing 'well-established and standardized'
treatment techniques with specific indications for their use, it has
probably come closest to this goal with the systematic desensitization
of isolated phobias. However, there is also evidence that behaviour
therapy can have a significant beneficial effect in more complex

236

neurotic and personality disturbances. Psychiatric departments which have behaviour therapists find they can make a valuable contribution to therapy and research.

Research

With behaviour therapy in its present stage of development, and its limited number of therapists, the problem is posed of how best to use its resources. Should they concentrate their efforts on applying existing treatment methods or should the main emphasis be on research? Behaviour therapy is likely to remain of restricted value and fall into disrepute if further advances are not made or if it is uncritically and enthusiastically accepted as an efficacious treatment for a wide variety of psychiatric disorders. But even in our present state of knowledge, a number of criticisms can be made. Treatment programmes are often constructed without sufficient consideration of the existing relevant experimental data of learning and general psychology, with the result that the most effective learning procedures may not be employed. Once a particular treatment technique is selected, the therapist may ignore individual differences in the patient's reactions to treatment which should lead to a modification in the plan of treatment. Furthermore, the therapist's evaluation of the behavioural techniques at his command may lead to exclusive concentration on a narrow area of the patient's behaviour and so lead to inadequate and incomplete treatment.

It is worth bearing these points in mind when trying to elucidate the most fruitful areas of research. At present there is an urgent need to improve the efficacy and range of applicability of existing therapeutic methods. The most promising line of approach may come from the application of the findings of other branches of psychology including cognitive processes and social psychology in addition to learning theory. A less restricted aetiological orientation towards behaviour disorders is likely to result in more adequate treatment methods for the common psychiatric disorders. Some of the more experienced behaviour therapists are already adopting a broad spectrum approach directed at all the sources of maladaptive behaviour. Further improvement in treatment methods is likely to result from a more detailed study of patients who fail to respond to behaviour therapy.

Investigation of the variables determining failure could lead to the development of effective methods for their modification.

Although laboratory research is always essential and, for example, the isolated laboratory study of operant conditioning has already been of considerable value, it seems more likely that one of the more pressing problems encountered by the clinician will be resolved by clinical investigations directed towards the extension and generalization of therapeutic gains achieved in the hospital or clinic to everyday life. Useful advances may result from careful study of the individual patient in treatment. Specific hypotheses about the functional relationship between different symptoms can be made and tested by close observation of the changes in the symptoms during treatment.

Learning theorists have long given up the attempt to establish a single all-embracing theory of learning. Similarly, it would not be fruitful for behaviour therapists to become obsessed with designing 'crucial experiments' in an attempt to discover a single theory of behaviour change.

Large-scale clinical trials comparing the efficacy of behaviour therapy with other treatment methods do not seem to deserve priority at the moment. This is because behaviour techniques are still relatively new and are likely to undergo some modification before definitive techniques emerge. A disadvantage of this type of comparative trial at the present juncture is that methodological requirements necessitate fairly rigid control of the therapeutic procedures with the result that there is no chance to modify and improve the method of treatment during its course.

Training of behaviour therapists

The encouraging results and advances in the field of behaviour therapy have led to an increasing demand for behaviour therapists to work in a clinical research setting. At present, there is no formal training centre and the few places that accept a limited number of trainees are not adequately equipped and organized to provide suitable training. The pioneers in behaviour therapy were self taught and the majority of behaviour therapists of the new generation still have to acquire their skills as best they can. There is an urgent need for the establishment of good training centres.

The kind of training that a behaviour therapist requires is a matter of controversy and a lot of thinking and experimentation is still required before suitable training programmes can be constructed. Poser (1967) has recently discussed this topic and has suggested that two different levels of behaviour therapy training should be provided. The first-level training would be sufficient for personnel who would act as 'co-therapists'. Poser has in mind personnel such as nursing assistants and other hospital and occupational staff who would be able to carry out routine treatment techniques under supervision (see also Ayllon and Michael, 1959; Davison, 1965). For those wishing to become 'behaviour therapists', Poser suggests that formal training in clinical psychology or psychiatry would be required, and that such a training would enable them 'to take charge of behaviour therapy services and be responsible for the elaboration of treatment strategies for patients in his care'.

Behaviour therapy centres should be established within a setting where there is both wide access to the whole range of psychiatric disorders and where there is a chance that it can benefit from the mutual interchange of ideas and stimulation provided by other psychological and psychiatric approaches. Access to both academic departments of physiology, psychology and other behavioural sciences as well as clinical psychiatry would be beneficial. The actual training programme should take the form of an apprenticeship, with observation and demonstrations of treatment methods followed by the student assisting in and then conducting treatment under supervision. Poser suggests that the apprenticeship should be of six months' duration for co-therapists and four months' for those who are going on to train as behaviour therapists. This part of the course would consist of lectures and seminars on learning principles and their clinical application.

We would agree with Poser that neither sound theoretical and experimental knowledge nor clinical experience alone constitutes an adequate preparation for those wishing to apply behaviour therapy methods to psychiatric patients. Our own experience with the training of psychologists, clinical psychologists and psychiatrists for a minimum period of six months has emphasized the importance of both clinical experience and a knowledge of learning theory. Those with exclusively clinical or experimental psychology experience tend to

239

have more difficulty in training to be behaviour therapists. Laboratory investigation of some behavioural method, for example the desensitization of fear of animals in a selected sample of college students, does not automatically lead to expertise and proficiency in the application of behaviour therapy to clinical disorders.

A disadvantage of the training programme outlined by Poser is the implication that behaviour therapy procedures are easily taught and executed. In the absence of established routine procedures, this is not the case. Problems are frequently encountered during each session which require reassessment and modification of the treatment procedure. For these reasons it is questionable whether 'co-therapists' would have sufficient training for clinical work. It seems that the idea arose from some reports in which undergraduate students and hospital personnel, after a brief course of instruction, had been able to assist efficiently in research projects with volunteer subjects and operant technique programmes with ward patients. The behaviour therapist requires the kind of basic training suggested by Poser. But it is hard to visualize that a single course of training could be designed which would be of use for people with such different backgrounds as experimental psychology and clinical psychiatry. Psychiatrists are likely to have large gaps in their knowledge of learning and general psychology, while psychologists may be ignorant of the phenomenology of psychiatric disorder and inexperienced in the management of patients. Because of this, quite different courses of training will be required according to the students' previous experience.

Administration of behaviour therapy units

In discussing the difficulties which are encountered by behaviour therapists and psychiatrists in the clinical application of behaviour therapy, we would emphasize that they tend to arise from two main sources. One is the lack of communication and understanding between the staff involved in the care of the patient which can result in a perplexed patient receiving inconsistent management and incompatible methods of treatment. The second is the individual and often unpredicted course and response of the patient and his 'symptoms'. In our present state of knowledge, one cannot confidently account for these unexpected variations within the framework of learning theory in a manner which will automatically lead to a successful behavioural treatment method. These considerations indicate the need for behaviour therapists to work in close conjunction with psychiatrists, psychiatric social workers, nurses and occupational therapists so that a unified plan of treatment can be carried out. Another advantage of close co-operation between staff members with different orientations lies in the stimulation provided by the interchange of ideas and the opportunity afforded of employing a wider range of treatment methods. Apart from this, the need for medical assessment and availability of medical supervision during the treatment of patients has been discussed in the previous chapter. It seems, therefore, that clinical needs, as well as the requirements of research and teaching, are best met when behaviour therapy units are integrated within psychiatric departments so that patients and staff can benefit from the intercommunication, shared experience and the varied skills which are available.

References

ABRAHAM, K. (1911), 'Notes on the psychoanalytical investigation and treatment of manic depressive insanity and allied conditions', in *Selected Papers of Karl Abraham*, Hogarth Press, 1954.

AGRAS, W. S. (1965), 'An investigation of the decrement of anxiety responses during systematic desensitization therapy', *Behav. Res. Ther.*, vol. 2, pp. 267–70.

AGRAS, W. S. (1967), 'Transfer during systematic desensitization therapy', *Behav. Res. Ther.*, vol. 5, pp. 193–9.

AGRAS, W. S., LEITENBERG, H., and BARLOW, D. H. (1968), 'Social reinforcement in the modification of agoraphobia', *Arch. gen. Psychiat.*, vol. 19, pp. 423 7.

ALEXANDER, F. (1963), 'The dynamics of psychotherapy in the light of learning theory', *Amer. J. Psychiat.*, vol. 120, pp. 440–48.

ALEXANDER, F., and FRENCH, M. T. (1946), *Psychoanalytic Therapy*, Ronald Press.

ANANT, S. (1968), 'Comment on a follow-up of alcoholics', *Behav. Res. Ther.*, vol. 6, p. 133.

ANDREWS, G., HARRIS, M., GARSIDE, R., and KAY, D. (1964), *The Syndrome of Stuttering*, Heinemann Medical Books.

ARONFREED, J., and REBER, A. (1965), 'Internalised behavioral suppression and the timing of social punishment', *J. Personal. soc. Psychol.*, vol. 1, pp. 3–16.

ASHEM, B., and DONNER, L. (1968), 'Covert sensitization with alcoholics', *Behav. Res. Ther.*, vol. 6, pp. 7–12.

ATTHOWE, J. M., and KRASNER, L. (1968), 'Preliminary report on the application of contingent reinforcement procedures (token economy) on a "chronic" psychiatric ward', *J. abnorm. soc. Psychol.*, vol. 73, pp. 37–43.

AYLLON, T. (1963), 'Intensive treatment of psychotic behaviour by stimulus satiation and food reinforcement', *Behav. Res. Ther.*, vol. 1, pp. 53–62.

AYLLON, T., and AZRIN, N. H. (1964), 'Reinforcement and instructions with mental patients', *J. exp. Anal. Behav.*, vol. 7, pp. 327–31.

AYLLON, T., and AZRIN, N. H. (1965), 'The measurement and reinforcement of behavior of psychotics', *J. exp. Anal. Behav.*, vol. 8, pp. 357–83.

References

AYLLON, T., and AZRIN, N. H. (1968), *The Token Economy: A
Motivational System for Therapy and Rehabilitation*, Appleton-Century-
Crofts.

AYLLON, T., and HAUGHTON, E. (1962), 'Control of the behavior of
schizophrenic patients by food', *J. exp. Anal. Behav.*, vol. 5, pp. 343–52.

AYLLON, T., and HAUGHTON, E. (1964), 'Modification of symptomatic
verbal behaviour of mental patients', *Behav. Res. Ther.*, vol. 2, pp. 87–97.

AYLLON, T., HAUGHTON, E., and HUGHES, H. B. (1965), 'Interpretation
of symptoms: fact or fiction', *Behav. Res. Ther.*, vol. 3, pp. 1–7.

AYLLON, T., and MICHAEL, J. (1959), 'The psychiatric nurse as a
behavioral engineer', *J. exp. Anal. Behav.*, vol. 3, pp. 323–34.

BACHRACH, A. J. (1964), 'Some applications of operant conditioning to
behavior therapy', in Wolpe, J., Salter, A., and Reyna, L. J. (eds.),
The Conditioning Therapies, Holt, Rinehart and Winston.

BACHRACH, A. J., ERWIN, W. J., and MOHR, J. P. (1965), 'The control
of eating behavior on an anorexic by operant conditioning techniques',
in Ullmann, L. P., and Krasner, L. (eds.), *Case Studies in Behavior
Modification*, Holt, Rinehart and Winston.

BADRI, M. B. (1967), 'A new technique for the systematic desensitization of
pervasive anxiety and phobic reactions', *J. Psychol.*, vol. 65, pp. 201–8.

BAER, D. M. (1962), 'Laboratory control of thumb-sucking in three young
children by withdrawal and representation of positive reinforcement',
J. exp. Anal. Behav., vol. 5, pp. 525–8.

BAER, D. M., and SHERMAN, J. A. (1964), 'Reinforcement control of
generalized imitation in young children', *J. exp. Child Psychol.*, vol. 1,
pp. 37–49.

BANCROFT, J., JONES, G. J., and PULLAN, B. R. (1966), 'A simple transducer
for measuring penile erection, with comments on its use in the treatment of
sexual disorders', *Behav. Res. Ther.*, vol. 4, pp. 239–41.

BANCROFT, J., and MARKS, I. (1968), 'Electric aversion therapy of sexual
deviations', *Proc. Roy. Soc. Med.*, vol. 61, pp. 796–9.

BANDURA, A. (1961), 'Psychotherapy as a learning process', *Psychol. Bull.*,
vol. 58, pp. 143–59.

BANDURA, A. (1965a), 'Behavioral modification through modeling
procedures', in Krasner, L., and Ullmann, L. P. (eds.), *Research in
Behavior Modification*, Holt, Rinehart and Winston.

BANDURA, A. (1965b), 'Vicarious processes: a case of no-trial learning',
in Berkowitz, L. (ed.), *Advances in Experimental Social Psychology*, vol. 2,
Academic Press.

BANDURA, A. (1968), 'Modeling approaches to the modification of phobic
disorders', in Porter, R. (ed.), *The Role of Learning in Psychotherapy*,
C.I.B.A. Foundation Symposium, Churchill.

BANDURA, A. (1969), *Principles of Behavior Modification*, Holt, Rinehart
and Winston.

BANDURA, A., BLANCHARD, E. D., and RITTER, B. J. (1968), 'The relative efficacy of desensitization and modeling approaches for inducing behavioral, affective and attitudinal dangers', unpublished manuscript, Stanford University.

BANDURA, A., GRUSEC, J. E., and MENLOVE, F. L. (1967), 'Vicarious extinction of avoidance behavior', *J. Personal. soc. Psychol.*, vol. 5, pp.16–23.

BANDURA, A., and MENLOVE, F. L. (1968), 'Factors determining vicarious extinction of avoidance behavior through symbolic modeling', *J. Personal. soc. Psychol.*, vol. 6, pp. 99–108.

BANDURA, A., and ROSENTHAL, T. L. (1966), 'Vicarious classical conditioning as a function of arousal level', *J. Personal. soc. Psychol.*, vol. 3, pp. 54–62.

BANDURA, A., and WALTERS, R. H. (1963), *Social Learning and Personality Development*, Holt, Rinehart and Winston.

BANNISTER, D., and MAIR, J. M. M. (1968), *The Evaluation of Personal Constructs*, Academic Press.

BARBER, T. X. (1965), 'Physiological effects of hypnotic suggestions', *Psychol. Bull.*, vol. 4, pp. 201–22.

BARKER, J. C. (1965), 'Behaviour therapy for transvestism: a comparison of pharmacological and electrical aversion techniques', *Brit. J. Psychiat.*, vol. 111, pp. 268–76.

BARLOW, D. H., LEITENBERG, H., AGRAS, W. S., and WINCZE, J. P. (1969), 'The transfer gap in systematice desensitization: an analogue study', *Behav. Res. Ther.*, vol. 7, pp. 191–6.

BARNETT, S. A. (1958), 'Physiological effects of social stress in wild rats', *J. psychosom. Res.*, vol. 3, pp. 1–11.

BARRETT, B. H. (1962), 'Reduction in rate of multiple tics by free operant conditioning methods', *J. nerv. ment. Dis.*, vol. 135, pp. 187–95.

BATESON, G., JACKSON, D. D., HALEY, J., and WEAKLAND, J. H. (1956), 'Towards a theory of schizophrenia', *Behav. Sci.*, vol. 1, pp. 251–64.

BECKER, W. C., and MATTESON, H. H. (1961), 'GSR conditioning, anxiety and extraversion', *J. abnorm. soc. Psychol.*, vol. 62, pp. 427–30.

BEECH, H. R. (1960), 'The symptomatic treatment of writer's cramp', in Eysenck, H. J. (ed.), *Behavioural Therapy and the Neuroses*, Pergamon Press.

BEECH, H. R. (1969), *Changing Man's Behaviour*, Penguin.

BEECHER, H. K. (1955), 'The powerful placebo', *Amer. Med. Assoc. J.*, vol. 159, pp. 1602–6.

BERGER, S. M. (1962), 'Conditioning through vicarious instigation', *Psychol. Rev.*, vol. 69, pp. 450–60.

BERGIN, A. E. (1967), 'Implications of psychotherapy research', *Int. J. Psychiat.*, vol. 3, pp. 136–50.

BERKSON, G. (1967), 'Abnormal stereotyped motor acts', in Zubin, J., and Hunt, H. F. (eds.), *Comparative Psychopathology: Animal and Human*, Grune and Stratton.

References

BERLYNE, D. E. (1960), *Conflict, Arousal and Curiosity*, McGraw-Hill.

BEVAN, W. (1964), 'Subliminal stimulation', *Psychol. Bull.*, vol. 61, pp. 81–99.

BIEBER, B., BIEBER, I., DAIN, H. J., DINCE, P. R., DRELLICH, M. G., GRAND, H. G., GRUNDLACH, R., KREMER, M. W., WILBUR, C. B., and BIEBER, T. B. (1962), *Homosexuality*, Basic Books.

BLACK, A. A. (1966), 'Factors predisposing to a placebo response in new out-patients with anxiety states', *Brit. J. Psychiat.*, vol. 112, pp. 557–67.

BLAKE, B. G. (1965), 'The application of behaviour therapy to the treatment of alcoholism', *Behav. Res. Ther.*, vol. 3, pp. 75–85.

BLAKE, B. G. (1967), 'A follow-up of alcoholics treated by behaviour therapy', *Behav. Res. Ther.*, vol. 5, pp. 89–94.

BLAKEMORE, C. B., THORPE, J. G., BARKER, J. C., CONWAY, C. G., and LAVIN, N. I. (1963), 'The application of faradic aversion conditioning to behaviour therapy in a case of transvestism', *Behav. Res. Ther.*, vol. 1, pp. 29–34.

BLEULER, E. (1950), *Dementia Praecox or the Group of Schizophrenias*, International Universities Press.

BOOKBINDER, L. (1962), 'Simple conditioning versus the dynamic approach to symptom and symptom substitution: a reply to Yates', *Psychol. Rev.*, vol. 10, pp. 71–7.

BOULOUGOURIS, J. C., and MARKS, I. M. (1969), 'Implosion (flooding) – a new treatment for phobias', *Brit. med. J.*, vol. 2, pp. 721–3.

BOWLBY, J. (1951), 'Maternal care and mental health', *W.H.O. Monograph Series*, no. 2, World Health Organization.

BOWLBY, J. (1961), 'Childhood mourning and its implications for psychiatry', *Amer. J. Psychiat.*, vol. 118, pp. 481–98.

BRADY, J. P. (1966), 'Brevital-relaxation treatment of frigidity', *Behav. Res. Ther.*, vol. 4, pp. 71–7.

BRADY, J. P. (1967), 'Comments on methohexitone-aided systematic desensitization', *Behav. Res. Ther.*, vol. 5, pp. 259–60.

BRADY, J. P., and LIND, D. L. (1961), 'Experimental analysis of hysterical blindness', *Arch. gen. Psychiat.*, vol. 4, pp. 331–9.

BRADY, J. V. (1957), 'A comparative approach to the experimental analysis of emotional behaviour', in Hoch, P. H., and Zubin, J. (eds.), *Experimental Psychopathology*, Grune and Stratton.

BRADY, J. V., PORTER, R. W., CONRAD, D. G., and MASON, J. W. (1958), 'Avoidance behavior and the development of gastroduodenal ulcers', *J. exp. Anal. Behav.*, vol. 1, pp. 69–72.

BREGER, L., and McGAUGH, J. (1965), 'Critique and reformulation of "learning theory" approaches to psychotherapy and neurosis', *Psychol. Bull.*, vol. 63, pp. 338–58.

BRIDGER, W. H., and MANDEL, I. J. (1964), 'A comparison of GSR responses produced by threat and electric shock', *J. psychiat. Res.*, vol. 2, pp. 31–40.

246

BRIDGER, W. H., and MANDEL, I. J. (1965), 'Cognitive expectancy and autonomic conditioning', in Wortis, J. (ed.), *Recent Advances in Biological Psychiatry*, vol. 7, Plenum Press.

BRIERLEY, H. (1967), 'The treatment of hysterical spasmodic torticollis by behaviour therapy', *Behav. Res. Ther.*, vol. 5, pp. 139–42.

BROADHURST, P. L. (1960), 'Abnormal animal behaviour', in Eysenck, H. J. (ed.), *Handbook of Abnormal Psychology*, Pitman.

BRODSKY, G. (1967), 'The relationship between verbal and non-verbal behaviour change', *Behav. Res. Ther.*, vol. 5, pp. 183–91.

BROGDEN, W. J. (1939), 'Sensory preconditioning', *J. exp. Psychol.*, vol. 25, pp. 323–32.

BROWN, J. S., KALISH, H. I., and FARBER, I. E. (1951), 'Conditioned fear as revealed by magnitude of startle response to an auditory stimulus', *J. exp. Psychol.*, vol. 41, pp. 317–28.

BROWNING, R. M. (1967), 'A same subject design for simultaneous comparison of three reinforcement contingencies', *Behav. Res. Ther.*, vol. 5, pp. 237–43.

BUEHLER, R. E., PATTERSON, G. R., and FURNISS, J. M. (1966), 'The reinforcement of behaviour in institutional settings', *Behav. Res. Ther.*, vol. 4, pp. 157–67.

BUGELSKI, R. (1938), 'Extinction with and without sub-goal reinforcement', *J. comp. Psychol.*, vol. 26, pp. 121–34.

BUNT, A. VAN DE, and BARENDREGT, J. T. (1961), 'Intercorrelations in three measures of conditioning', in Barendregt, J. T. (ed.), *Research in Psychodiagnostics*, Mouton, The Hague.

CAHOON, D. D. (1968), 'Symptom substitution and the behaviour therapies: a reappraisal', *Psychol. Bull.*, vol. 69, pp. 149–56.

CAMPBELL, D., SANDERSON, R. E., and LAVERTY, S. G. (1964), 'Characteristics of a conditioned response in human subjects during extinction trials following a single traumatic conditioning trial', *J. abnorm. soc. Psychol.*, vol. 68, pp. 627–39.

CASE, H. W. (1960), 'Therapeutic methods in stuttering and speech blocking', in Eysenck, H. J. (ed.), *Behaviour Therapy and the Neuroses*, Pergamon Press.

CAUTELA, J. R. (1966), 'Treatment of compulsive behaviour by covert sensitization', *Psychol. Rec.*, vol. 16, pp. 33–41.

CAUTELA, J. R. (1967), 'Covert desensitization', *Psychol. Rep.*, vol. 20, pp. 459–68.

CHAPMAN, J. (1966), 'The early symptoms of schizophrenia', *Brit. J. Psychiat.*, vol. 112, pp. 225–7.

CHERRY, C., and SAYERS, B. McA. (1956), 'Experiments upon the total inhibition of stammering by external control and some clinical results', *J. psychosom. Res.*, vol. 1, pp. 233–46.

CHURCH, R. M. (1963), 'The varied effects of punishment on behaviour', *Psychol. Rev.*, vol. 70, pp. 369–402.

References

CLARK, D. F. (1966), 'Behaviour therapy of Gilles de la Tourette's syndrome', *Brit. J. Psychiat.*, vol. 112, pp. 771–8.

CLARKE, J. R. (1953), 'The effect of fighting on the adrenals, thymus and spleen of the vole', *J. Endocrin.*, vol. 9, pp. 114–26.

COLE, S. N., and SIPPRELLE, C. N. (1967), 'Extinction of a classically conditioned GSR as a function of awareness', *Behav. Res. Ther.*, vol. 5, pp. 331–7.

CONGER, J. J. (1956), 'Reinforcement theory and the dynamics of alcoholism', *Q. J. Stud. Alcohol.*, vol. 17, pp. 296–305.

COOKE, G. (1966), 'The efficacy of two desensitization procedures: an analogue study,' *Behav. Res. Ther.*, vol. 4, pp. 17–24.

COOKE, G. (1968), 'Evaluation of the efficacy of the components of reciprocal inhibition psychotherapy', *J. abnorm. Psychol.*, vol. 73, pp. 464–7.

COOPER, J. E. (1963), 'A study of behaviour therapy in thirty psychiatric patients', *Lancet*, vol. 1, pp. 411–15.

COOPER, J. E., GELDER, M. G., and MARKS, I. M. (1965), 'Results of behaviour therapy in 77 psychiatric patients', *Brit. med. J.*, vol. 1, pp. 1222–5.

CRISP, A. H. (1966), ' "Transference", "symptom emergence" and "social repercussion" in behaviour therapy', *Brit. J. med. Psychol.*, vol. 39, pp. 179–96.

CROSBY, N. D. (1950), 'Essential enuresis: successful treatment based on physiological concepts', *Med. J. Aust.*, vol. 2, pp. 533–43.

DAVIDSON, P. O., PAYNE, R. W., and SLOANE, R. B. (1964), 'Introversion, neuroticism and conditioning', *J. abnorm. soc. Psychol.*, vol. 68, pp. 136–43.

DAVIDSON, P. O., PAYNE, R. W., and SLOANE, R. B. (1966), 'Cortical inhibition, drive level and conditioning', *J. abnorm. soc. Psychol.*, vol. 71, pp. 310–14.

DAVIES, D. L., SHEPPARD, M., and MEYERS, E. (1956), 'The two year prognosis of fifty alcoholic addicts after treatment in hospital', *Q. J. Stud. Alcohol.*, vol. 17, pp. 485–502.

DAVISON, G. C. (1964), 'A social learning therapy programme with an autistic child', *Behav. Res. Ther.*, vol. 2, pp. 149–59.

DAVISON, G. C. (1965), 'The training of undergraduates as social reinforcers for autistic children', in Ullmann, L. P., and Krasner, L. (eds.), *Case Studies in Behavior Modification*, Holt, Rinehart and Winston.

DAVISON, G. C. (1966), 'Anxiety under total curarization: implications for the role of muscular relaxation in the desensitization of neurotic fears', *J. nerv. ment. Dis.*, vol. 143, pp. 443–8.

DAVISON, G. C. (1967), 'Some problems of logic and conceptualization in behavior therapy research and theory', paper read at Symposium on Behavior Therapy from the Scientist–Practitioner Point of View, 75th Annual Convention of American Psychological Association, September.

DAVISON, G. C. (1968a), 'Elimination of a sadistic fantasy by a client-controlled counterconditioning technique: a case study', *J. abnorm. soc. Psychol.*, vol. 73, pp. 84–90.

DAVISON, G. C. (1968b), 'Self-control in an unruly young adolescent through imaginal aversive contingency and one-downmanship', unpublished manuscript, State University of New York.

DAVISON, G. C., (1968c), 'Systematic desensitization as a counterconditioning process', *J. abnorm. soc. Psychol.*, vol. 73, pp. 91–9.

DAVISON, G. C. (1969), 'Appraisal of behavior modification techniques with adults in institutional settings', in Franks, C. M. (ed.), *Behavior Therapy: Appraisal and Status*, McGraw-Hill.

DAVISON, G. C., and VALINS, S. (1968), 'On self-produced and drug-produced relaxation', *Behav. Res. Ther.*, vol. 6, pp. 401–2.

DEKKER, E., and GROEN, J. (1956), 'Reproducible psychogenic attacks of asthma', *J. psychosom. Res.*, vol. 1, pp. 58–67.

DELUDE, L. A., and CARLSON, N. J. (1964), 'A test of the conservation of anxiety and partial irreversibility hypotheses', *Canad. J. Psychol.*, vol. 18, pp. 15–22.

DENKER, P. G. (1947), 'Results of treatment of psychoneuroses by the general practitioner: a follow-up study of 500 cases', *Arch. Neurol. Psychiat.*, vol. 57, pp. 504–5.

DENNEHY, C. M. (1966), 'Childhood bereavement and psychiatric illness', *Brit. J. Psychiat.*, vol. 112, pp. 1049–69.

DICARA, L. V., and MILLER, N. E. (1968), 'Changes in heart rate instrumentally learned by curarized rats as avoidance responses', *J. comp. physiol. Psychol.*, vol. 65., pp. 8–12.

DITTIES, J. E. (1957a), 'Extinction during psychotherapy of GSR accompanying embarrassing statements', *J. aborm. soc. Psychol.*, vol. 54, pp. 187–91.

DITTIES, J. E. (1957b), 'Galvanic skin responses as a measure of patient's reaction to therapist's permissiveness', *J. abnorm. soc. Psychol.*, vol. 55, pp. 295–303.

DOLLARD, J., and MILLER, N. E. (1950), *Personality and Psychotherapy*, McGraw-Hill.

DONNER, L., and GUERNEY, B. G. (1969), 'Automated group desensitization for test anxiety', *Behav. Res. Ther.*, vol. 7, pp. 1–13.

DUNLAP, K. (1932), *Habits, Their Making and Unmaking*, Liveright.

EFRON, R. (1957), 'The conditioned inhibition of uncinate fits', *Brain*, vol. 80, pp. 251–62.

ENGEL, G. L. (1962), *Psychological Development in Health and Disease*, Saunders.

ERIKSEN, C. W. (1958), 'Unconscious processes', in Jones, M. R. (ed.), *Nebraska Symposium of Motivation*, Nebraska University Press.

References

ERIKSON, E. H. (1965), *Childhood and Society*, 2nd edn, Hogarth Press.

ESTES, W. K. (1944), 'An experimental study of punishment', *Psychol. Monogr.*, vol. 57, no. 3, whole no. 363.

EVANS, I., and WILSON, T. (1968), 'Note on the terminological confusion surrounding systematic desensitization', *Psychol. Rep.*, vol. 22, pp. 187–91.

EYSENCK, H. J. (1957), *Dynamics of Anxiety and Hysteria*, Routledge and Kegan Paul.

EYSENCK, H. J. (ed.) (1960a), *Behaviour Therapy and the Neuroses*, Pergamon Press.

EYSENCK, H. J. (1960b), 'The effects of psychotherapy', in Eysenck, H. J. (ed.), *Handbook of Abnormal Psychology*, Pitman.

EYSENCK, H. J. (1963a), 'Behaviour therapy, extinction and relapse', *Brit. J. Psychiat.*, vol. 109, pp. 12–18.

EYSENCK, H. J. (1963b), 'Behavior therapy, spontaneous remission and transference in neurotics', *Amer. J. Psychiat.*, vol. 119, pp. 867–71.

EYSENCK, H. J. (ed.) (1964), *Experiments in Behaviour Therapy*, Pergamon Press.

EYSENCK, H. J. (1965), 'Extraversion and the acquisition of eyeblink and GSR conditioned response', *Psychol. Bull.*, vol. 63, pp. 258–70.

EYSENCK, H. J. (1968a), 'A theory of the incubation of anxiety fear responses', *Behav. Res. Ther.*, vol. 6, pp. 309–21.

EYSENCK, H. J. (1968b), *The Biological Basis of Behavior*, Thomas.

EYSENCK, H. J., and EYSENCK, S. B. G. (1964), *Manual of the Eysenck Personality Inventory*, London University Press.

EYSENCK, H. J., and RACHMAN, S. (1965), *The Causes and Cures of Neurosis*, Routledge and Kegan Paul.

FAIRWEATHER, G. W. (ed.) (1964), *Social Psychology in Treating Mental Illness*, Wiley.

FAIRWEATHER, G. W., SANDERS, D. H., MAYNARD, H., and CRESSLER, D.L. (1969), *Community Life for the Mentally Ill*, Aldine, cited by BANDURA (1969).

FARRAR, C. H., POWELL, B. J., and MARTIN, L. K. (1968), 'Punishment of alcohol consumption by apneic paralysis', *Behav. Res. Ther.*, vol. 6, pp. 13–16.

FEATHER, B. W. (1965), 'Semantic generalization of classically conditioned responses: a review', *Psychol. Bull.*, vol. 63, pp. 425–41.

FELDMAN, M. P. (1966), 'Aversion therapy for sexual deviations: a critical review', *Psychol. Bull.*, vol. 65, pp. 65–9.

FELDMAN, M. P., and MacCULLOCH, M. J. (1965), 'The application of anticipatory avoidance learning to the treatment of homosexuality. 1: Theory, techniques and preliminary results', *Behav. Res. Ther.*, vol. 2, pp. 165–83.

FENICHEL, O. (1946), *The Psychoanalytic Theory of Neurosis*, Routledge and Kegan Paul.

FERSTER, C. B. (1961), 'Positive reinforcement and behavioural deficits in autistic children', *Child Develop.*, vol. 32, pp. 437–56.

FERSTER, C. B. (1965), 'Classification of behavioral pathology', in Ullmann, L. P., and Krasner, L. (eds.), *Research in Behavior Modification*, Holt, Rinehart and Winston.

FERSTER, C. B., and SKINNER B. F. (1957), *Schedules of Reinforcement*, Appleton-Century-Crofts.

FIELD, E. (1967), *A Validation Study of Hewitt and Jenkins' Hypothesis*, Home Office Research Unit Report, no. 10, H.M.S.O.

FISH, H. J. (1964), *An Outline of Psychiatry*, Wright.

FLUGEL, J. C. (1945), *Man, Morals and Society*, Duckworth.

FOLKINS, C. H., LAWSON, K. D., OPTON, E. M., and LAZURUS, R. S. (1968), 'Densensitization and the experimental reduction of threat', *J. abnorm. Psychol.*, vol. 73, pp. 100–113.

FONBERG, E. (1956), 'On the manifestation of conditioned defensive reactions in stress', in Wolpe, J. (ed.) (1958), *Psychotherapy by Reciprocal Inhibition*, Stanford University Press.

FOWLER, R. L., and KIMMEL, H. D. (1962), 'Operant conditioning of the GSR', *J. exp. Psychol.*, vol. 63, pp. 563–7.

FRANK, J. D. (1961), *Persuasion and Healing*, Johns Hopkins Press.

FRANK, J. D. (1968), 'The role of hope in psychotherapy', *Int. J. Psychiat.*, vol. 5, pp. 383–400.

FRANK, J. D., NASH, E. H., STONE, A. R., and IMBER, S. D. (1962), 'Immediate and long-term symptomatic course of psychiatric out-patients', *Amer. J. Psychiat.*, vol. 120, pp. 429–39.

FRANKS, C. M. (1960), 'Conditioning and abnormal behaviour', in Eysenck, H. J. (ed.), *Handbook of Abnormal Psychology*, Pitman.

FRANKS, C. M. (1966), 'Conditioning and conditioned aversion therapies in the treatment of the alcoholics', *Int. J. Addict.*, vol. 1, pp. 62–98.

FRANKS, C. M., and TROUTON, D. S. (1958), 'The effects of amobarbital sodium and dexamphetamine sulphate on the conditioning of the eyeblink response', *J. comp. physiol. Psychol.*, vol. 51, pp. 220–22.

FRANSELLA, F. (1967), 'Rhythm as a distractor in the modification of stuttering', *Behav. Res. Ther.*, vol. 5, pp. 253–5.

FRANSELLA, F., and BEECH, H. R. (1965), 'An experimental analysis of the effect of rhythm on the speech of stutterers', *Behav. Res. Ther.*, vol. 3, pp. 195–201.

FRAZIER, T. W. (1966), 'Avoidance conditioning of heart rate in humans', *Psychophys.*, vol. 3, pp. 188–202.

FREEMAN, H. S., and KENDRICK, D. C. (1960), 'A case of cat phobia', *Brit. med. J.*, vol. 2, pp. 497–502.

FREUD, S. (1909), *Studies on Hysteria*, in standard edition of *Complete Psychological Works*, vol. 2, Hogarth Press.

References

FREUD, S. (1917), *Mourning and Melancholia*, in standard edition of *Complete Psychological Works*, vol. 14 (1957), Hogarth Press.

FREUD, S. (1918), *Totem and Taboo*, in standard edition of *Complete Psychological Works*, vol. 13 (1955), Hogarth Press.

FREUD, S. (1937), *Analysis Terminable and Interminable*, in standard edition of *Complete Psychological Works*, vol. 23 (1964), Hogarth Press.

FREUD, S. (1940), *An Outline of Psychoanalysis*, in standard edition of *Complete Psychological Works*, vol. 23 (1964), Hogarth Press.

FREUND, K. (1960), 'Some problems in the treatment of homosexuality', in Eysenck, H. J. (ed.), *Behaviour Therapy and the Neuroses*, Pergamon Press.

FRIED, R. (1967), 'Essentials of electroshock and electroshock devices', *Newsletter*, Assoc. Advance Behav. Ther., vol. 2, no. 2, pp. 3–4.

FRIEDMAN, D. (1966a), 'A new technique for the systematic desensitization of phobic symptoms', *Behav. Res. Ther.*, vol. 4, pp. 139–40.

FRIEDMAN, D. (1966b), 'Treatment of a case of dog phobia in a deaf mute by behaviour therapy', *Behav. Res. Ther.*, vol. 4, p. 141.

FRIEDMAN, D. E. I., and SILVERSTONE, J. T. (1967), 'Treatment of phobic patients by systematic desensitization', *Lancet*, vol. 1, pp. 470–72.

FRIEDMAN, H. J. (1963), 'Patient expectancy and symptom reduction', *Arch. gen. Psychiat.*, vol. 8, pp. 61–7.

FURNEAUX, W. D., and GIBSON, H. B. (1961), 'A children's personality inventory designed to measure neuroticism and extraversion', *Brit. J. educ. Psychol.*, vol. 31, pp. 204–7.

GALAMBOS, R., and MORGAN, C. T. (1960), 'The neural basis of learning', in *Handbook of Physiology*, vol. 3, *Neurophysiology*, section 1, American Physiological Society.

GALAMBOS, R., and SHEATZ, G. S. (1962), 'An EEG study of classical conditioning', *Amer. J. Physiol.*, vol. 203, pp. 173–84.

GALE, D. S., STRUMFELS, G., and GALE, E. (1966), 'A comparison of reciprocal inhibition and experimental extinction in the psychotherapeutic process', *Behav. Res. Ther.*, vol. 4, pp. 149–55.

GANTT, W. H. (1953), 'Principles of nervous breakdown: schizokinesis and autokinesis', *Ann. N.Y. Acad. Sci.*, vol. 56, pp. 143–63.

GAMBRILL, E. (1967), 'Effectiveness of the counterconditioning procedure in eliminating avoidance behaviour', *Behav. Res. Ther.*, vol. 5, pp. 263–73.

GARFIELD, Z. A., DARWIN, P. L., SINGER, B. A., and McBREARTY, J. F. (1967), 'Effect of "in vivo" training on experimental desensitization of a phobia', *Psychol. Rep.*, vol. 20, pp. 515–19.

GEER, J. H. (1965), 'The development of a scale to measure fear', *Behav. Res. Ther.*, vol. 3, pp. 45–53.

GELDER, M. G. (1968), 'Desensitization and psychotherapy research, *Brit. J. med. Psychol.*, vol. 41, pp. 39–46.

References

GELDER, M. G., and MARKS, I. M. (1966), 'Severe agoraphobia: a controlled prospective trial of behaviour therapy,' *Brit. J. Psychiat.*, vol. 112, pp. 309–19.

GELDER, M. G., and MARKS, I. M. (1968), 'Desensitization and phobias: a crossover study', *Brit. J. Psychiat.*, vol. 114, pp. 323–8.

GELDER, M. G., MARKS, I. M., WOLFF, H. E., and CLARKE, M. (1967), 'Desensitization and psychotherapy in the treatment of phobic states: a controlled inquiry', *Brit. J. Psychiat.*, vol. 113, pp. 53–73.

GELDER, M. G., and MATHEWS, A. M. (1968), 'Forearm blood flow and phobic anxiety', *Brit. J. Psychiat.*, vol. 114, pp. 1371–6.

GELFAND, D. M., GELFELAND, S., and DOBSON, W. R. (1967), 'Unprogrammed reinforcement of patients' behaviour in a mental hospital', *Behav. Res. Ther.*, vol. 5, pp. 201–7.

GENERAL REGISTER OFFICE (1968), *A Glossary of Mental Disorders*, Studies on Medical and Population Subjects, no. 22, H.M.S.O.

GERICKE, O. L. (1965), 'Practical use of operant conditioning procedures in a mental hospital', *Psychiat. Stud. Proj.*, vol. 3, pp. 1–10.

GLASER, E. N. (1966), *The Physiological Basis of Habituation*, Oxford University Press.

GLATT, M. M. (1961), 'Treatment results in an English mental hospital alcoholic unit', *Acta Psychiatrica Scandinavica*, vol. 37, pp. 143–68.

GLEITMAN, H., NACHMIAS, J., and NEISSER, U. (1954), 'The s–r reinforcement theory of extinction', *Psychol. Rev.*, vol. 61, pp. 23–33.

GOLD, S., and NEUFELD, I. L. (1965), 'A learning approach to the treatment of homosexuality', *Behav. Res. Ther.*, vol. 2, pp. 201–4.

GOLDIAMOND, I. (1965), 'Stuttering and fluency as manipulatable operant response classes', in Krasner, L., and Ullmann, L. P. (eds.), *Research in Behavior Modification*, Holt, Rinehart and Winston.

GOLDSTEIN, A. P. (1960), 'Patients' expectancies and non-specific therapy as a basis for (un)spontaneous remission', *J. clin. Psychol.*, vol. 16, pp. 399–403.

GOLDSTEIN, A. P. (1962), *Therapist–Patient Expectancies in Psychotherapy*, Pergamon Press.

GOLDSTEIN, A. P. (1968), 'Maximizing expectancy effects in psychotherapeutic practice', *Int. J. Psychiat.*, vol. 5, pp. 397–400.

GOLDSTEIN, A. P., HELLER, K., and SECHREST, L. B. (1966), *Psychotherapy and the Psychology of Behavior Change*, Holt, Rinehart and Winston.

GOTTSCHALK, L. A., and AUERBACH, A. H. (eds.) (1966), *Methods of Research in Psychotherapy*, Appleton-Century-Crofts.

GRANVILLE-GROSSMAN, K. L. (1968), 'The early environment in affective disorders', in Coppen, A., and Walk, A. (eds.), *Recent Developments in Affective Disorders*, *Brit. J. Psychiat.*, Special Publication, no. 2, Royal Medico-Psychological Association.

GREENSPOON, J. (1962), 'Verbal conditioning and clinical psychology', in Bachrach, A. J. (ed.), *Experimental Foundations in Clinical Psychology*, Basic Books.

253

References

GREENWALD, A. G. (1965), 'Punishment as a means of increasing the "strength" of a response', paper presented at the Annual Meeting of the Eastern Psychological Association.

GREER, H. S., and CAWLEY, R. H. (1966), *Natural History of Neurotic Illness*, Australian Medical Publishing Co.

GRINKER, R. R., and SPIEGEL, J. P. (1945), *Men Under Stress*, Blakiston.

GROSSBERG, J. M., and WILSON, H. K. (1965), 'A correlational comparison of the Wolpe-Lang Fear Survey Schedule and Taylor Manifest Anxiety Scale', *Behav. Res. Ther.*, vol. 3, pp. 125–8.

GUTHRIE, E. R. (1935), *The Psychology of Learning*, Harper.

GWINN, G. T. (1949), 'The effect of punishment on acts motivated by fear', *J. exp. Psychol.*, vol. 39, pp. 260–69.

HAGMAN, C. (1932), 'A study of fears of children in the pre-school age', *J. exp. Psychol.*, vol. 1, pp. 110–30.

HAIN, J. D., BUTCHER, R. H. G., and STEVENSON, I. (1966), 'Systematic desensitization therapy: an analysis of results in twenty-seven patients', *Brit. J. Psychiat.*, vol. 112, pp. 295–307.

HARLOW, H. F. (1963), 'The maternal affectional system', in Foss, B. M. (ed.), *Determinants of Infant Behaviour*, Methuen.

HARTMANN, H. (1964), *Essays on Ego Psychology*, Hogarth Press.

HAWKINS, R. P., PETERSON, R. F., SCHWEID, E., and BIJON, S. W. (1966), 'Behaviour therapy at home: amelioration of problem parent–child reactions with the parent in a therapeutic role', *J. exp. Child Psychol.*, vol. 4, pp. 99–107.

HEAP, R. F., and SIPPRELLE, C. N. (1966), 'Extinction as a function of insight', *Psychotherapy*, vol. 3, pp. 81–4.

HEBB, D. O. (1947), 'Spontaneous neurosis in chimpanzees: theoretical relationships with clinical and experimental phenomena', *Psychosom. Med.*, vol. 9, pp. 3–19.

HEBB, D. O. (1955), 'Drives and the C.N.S.', *Psychol. Rev.*, vol. 62, pp. 243–54.

HEBB, D. O. (1958), 'Alice in Wonderland or psychology among the biological sciences', in Harlow, H. F., and Woolsey, C. N. (eds.), *Biological and Biochemical Bases of Behavior*, Wisconsin University Press.

HEFFERLINE, R. F. (1962), 'Learning theory and clinical psychology – an eventual symbiosis?', in Bachrach, A. J. (ed.), *Experimental Foundations of Clinical Psychology*, Basic Books.

HEWITT, J., and JENKINS, R. L. (1946), *Fundamental Patterns of Maladjustment*, Michigan Child Guidance Institute.

HILGARD, E. R., and MARQUIS, D. M. (1940), *Conditioning and Learning*, Appleton-Century-Crofts.

HINDE, R. A. (1960), 'An ethological approach', in Tanner, J. M. (ed.), *Stress and Psychiatric Disorder*, Blackwell.

HOBBS, N. (1962), 'Sources of gain in psychotherapy', *Amer. Psychol.*, vol. 17, pp. 741–7.

HOCUTT, M. (1967), 'On the alleged circularity of Skinner's concept of stimulus', *Psychol. Rev.*, vol. 74, pp. 530–32.

HOEHN-SARIC, R., FRANK, J. D., IMBER, S. D., NASH, E. H., STONE, A. R., and BATTLE, C. C. (1965), 'Systematic preparation of patients for psychotherapy', *J. Psychiat. Res.*, vol. 2, pp. 267–81.

HOENIG, J., and REED, G. F. (1966), 'The objective assessment of desensitization', *Brit. J. Psychiat.*, v 1. 112, pp. 1279–83.

HOGAN, R. A. (1966), 'Implosive therapy in the short-term treatment of psychotics', *Psychother.*, vol. 3, pp. 25–32.

HOGAN, R. A., and KIRCHNER, J. H. (1967), 'Preliminary reports of the extinction of learned fears via short-term implosive therapy', *J. abnorm. Psychol.*, vol. 72, pp. 106–9.

HOGAN, R. A., and KIRCHNER, J. H. (1968), 'Implosive, eclectic verbal, and bibliotherapy in the treatment of fears of snakes', *Behav. Res. Ther.*, vol. 6, pp. 167–71.

HOLLAND, J. G., and SKINNER, B. F. (1961), *The Analysis of Behaviour*, McGraw-Hill.

HOLT, R. R. (1967), 'Ego autonomy re-evaluated', *Int. J. Psychiat.*, vol. 3, pp. 481–503.

HOLZ, W. C., and AZRIN, N. H. (1961), 'Discrimination properties of punishment', *J. exp. Anal. Behav.*, vol. 4, pp. 225–32.

HOMME, L. (1965), 'Perspective in psychology. 24. Control of coverants, the operants of the mind', *Psychol. Rec.*, vol. 15, pp. 501–11.

HONIGFELD, G. (1964), 'Non-specific factors in treatment: 1. Review of placebo reactions and placebo reactors. 2. Review of socio-psychological factors', *Dis. nerv. Syst.*, vol. 25, pp. 135–56, 225–39.

HSU, J. J. (1965), 'Electroconditioning therapy of alcoholics: a preliminary report', *Q. J. Stud. Alcohol.*, vol. 26, pp. 449–59.

HUDSON, B. B. (1950), 'One trial learning in the domestic rat', *Genet. Psychol. Monogr.*, pp. 94–146.

HULL, C. L. (1943), *Principles of Behavior*, Appleton-Century-Crofts.

HULL, C. L. (1952), *A Behavior System*, Yale University Press.

HUNT, H. F. (1961), 'Methods for studying the behavioral effects of drugs', *Ann. Rev. Pharmacol.*, vol. 1, pp. 125–44.

HUSSAIN, A. (1964), 'The results of behavior therapy in 105 cases', in Wolpe, J., Salter, A., and Reyna, J. (eds.), *Conditioning Therapies*, Holt, Rinehart and Winston.

INGRAM, I. M. (1961), 'The obsessional personality and obsessional illnesses', *Amer. J. Psychiat.*, vol. 117, pp. 1016–19.

ISAACS, W., THOMAS, J., and GOLDIAMOND, I. (1960), 'Application of operant conditioning to reinstate verbal behaviour in psychotics', *J. Speech Hearing Disord.*, vol. 25, pp. 8–12.

JACOBSON, E. (1938), *Progressive Relaxation*, Chicago University Press.

JACOBSON, E. (1964), *Anxiety and Tension Control*, Lipincott.

References

JASPERS, K. (1963), *General Psychopathology*, Manchester University Press.

JERSILD, A. T., and HOLMES, F. B. (1935), 'Children's fears', *J. Psychol.*, vol. 1, pp. 75–104.

JONES, H. G. (1956), 'The application of conditioning and learning techniques to the treatment of a psychiatric patient', *J. abnorm. soc. Psychol.*, vol. 52, pp. 414–20.

JONES, H. G. (1960), 'The behavioural treatment of enuresis nocturna', in Eysenck, H. J., (ed.), *Behaviour Therapy and the Neuroses*, Pergamon Press.

JONES, M. C. (1924a), 'The elimination of children's fear', *J. exp. Psychol.*, vol. 7, pp. 383–90.

JONES, M. C. (1924b), 'A laboratory study of fear: the case of Peter', *Pedagog. Semin.*, vol. 31, pp. 308–15.

JOYCE, C. R. B. (1962), 'Differences between physicians as revealed by clinical trials', *Proc. Roy. Soc. Med.*, vol. 55, pp. 776–8.

JUNG, C. J. (1960), *The Psychogenesis of Mental Disease*, Routledge and Kegan Paul.

KAHANE, M. (1955), 'An experimental investigation of a conditioning treatment and a preliminary study of the psycho-analytic theory of the etiology of nocturnal enuresis', *Amer. Psychol.*, vol. 10, pp. 369–70.

KANFER, F. H. (1961), 'Comments on learning in psychotherapy', *Psychol. Rep.*, vol. 9, pp. 681–99.

KARDINER, A., KARUSH, A., and OVESY, L. (1959), 'A methodological study of Freudian theory', *J. nerv. ment. Dis.*, vol. 129, pp. 11–19, 133–43, 207–21, 341–56.

KATKIN, E. S., and MURRAY, E. N. (1968), 'Instrumental conditioning of autonomically mediated behaviour: theoretical and methodological issues', *Psychol. Bull.*, vol. 70, pp. 52–68.

KELLNER, R. (1967), 'The evidence in favour of psychotherapy', *Brit. J. med. Psychol.*, vol. 40, pp. 341–58.

KELLY, D. H. (1966), 'Measurement of anxiety by forearm blood flow', *Brit. J. Psychiat.*, vol. 112, pp. 789–98.

KELLY, D., and MARTIN, I. (1969), 'Autonomic reactivity, eyelid conditioning and their relationship to neuroticism and extraversion', *Behav. Res. Ther.*, vol. 7, pp. 233–44.

KELLY, D. H. W., and WALTER, C. J. S. (1968), 'The relationship between clinical diagnosis and anxiety, assessed by forearm blood flow and other measurements', *Brit. J. Psychiat.*, vol. 114, pp. 611–26.

KELLY, G. A. (1955), *The Psychology of Personal Constructs*, Norton.

KENDALL, R. E. (1968), 'The problem of classification', in *Recent Developments in Affective Disorders*, *Brit. J. Psychiat.*, Special Bull., Royal Medico-Psychological Association.

KENDALL, R. E., and STATON, M. C. (1965), 'The fate of untreated alcoholics', *Q. J. Stud. Alcohol.*, vol. 26, pp. 685–6.

256

KENNEDY, T. (1964), 'Treatment of chronic schizophrenia by behaviour therapy: case reports', *Behav. Res. Ther.*, vol. 2, pp. 1–6.

KIESLER, D. J. (1966), 'Some myths of psychotherapy research and the search for a paradigm', *Psychol. Bull.*, vol. 65, pp. 110–36.

KIMBLE, G. (1961), *Hilgard and Marquis' 'Conditioning and Learning'*, Appleton-Century-Crofts.

KIMBLE, G. (1967), *Foundations of Conditioning and Learning*, Appleton-Century-Crofts.

KIMBLE, G., and KENDALL, J. (1953), 'A comparison of two methods of producing experimental extinction', *J. exp. Psychol.*, vol. 45, pp. 87–9.

KING, G. F., ARMITAGE, S. G., and TILTON, J. R. (1960), 'A therapeutic approach to schizophrenics of extreme pathology', *J. abnorm. soc. Psychol.*, vol. 61, pp. 276–86.

KIRK, R. V. (1968), 'Perceptual defect and role handicap: missing links in explaining the aetiology of schizophrenia', *Brit. J. Psychiat.*, vol. 114, pp. 1509–21.

KNOWLES, J. B. (1963), 'Conditioning and the placebo effect: the effects of decaffeinated coffee on simple reaction time in habitual coffee drinkers', *Behav. Res. Ther.*, vol. 1, pp. 151–7.

KOENIG, K. P., and MASTERS, J. (1965), 'Experimental treatment of habitual smoking', *Behav. Res. Ther.*, vol. 3, pp. 235–43.

KOLVIN, I. (1967), ' "Aversion imagery" treatment in adolescents', *Behav. Res. Ther.*, vol. 5, pp. 245–8.

KONDAS, O. (1967a), 'Reduction of examination anxiety and "stage-fright" by group desensitization and relaxation', *Behav. Res. Ther.*, vol. 5, pp. 275–81.

KONDAS, O. (1967b), 'The treatment of stammering in children by the shadowing method', *Behav. Res. Ther.*, vol. 5, pp. 325–9.

KRAFT, T. (1967), 'The use of methohexitone sodium in behaviour therapy', *Behav. Res. Ther.*, vol. 5, p. 257.

KRASNER, L. (1958), 'Studies of the conditioning of verbal behavior', *Psychol. Bull.*, vol. 55, pp. 148–70.

KRASNER, L. (1963), 'Reinforcement, verbal behavior and psychotherapy', *Amer. J. Orthopsychiat.*, vol. 33, pp. 601–13.

KRASNER, L. (1965), 'Verbal conditioning and psychotherapy', in Krasner, L., and Ullmann, L. P. (eds.), *Research in Behavior Modification*, Holt, Rinehart and Winston.

KRASNER, L. (1968), 'Assessment of token economy programmes in psychiatric patients', in Porter, R. (ed.), *The Role of Learning in Psychotherapy*, C.I.B.A. Foundation Symposium, Churchill.

KRASNOGORSKI, N. I. (1925), 'The conditioned reflexes and the children's neuroses', *Amer. J. Dis. Child.*, vol. 30, pp. 753–68.

KRASNOGORSKI, N. I. (1933), 'Physiology of cerebral activity in children as a new subject of pediatric investigation', *Amer. J. Dis. Child.*, vol. 46, pp. 473–94.

References

KRETSCHMER, E. (1934), *A Textbook of Medical Psychology*, trans. Strauss, E. B., Oxford University Press.

KUSHNER, M. (1967), 'Behavior therapy program of VA Hospital, Coral Gables, Florida', *Newsletter*, Assoc. Advance. Behav. Ther., vol. 2, no.1, p. 7.

LACEY, J. I., KAGAN, J., LACEY, B. L., and MOSS, H. A. (1963), 'The visceral level: situational determinants and behavioural correlates of autonomic response patterns', in Knapp, P. H. (ed.), *Expression of the Emotions of Man*, International Universities Press.

LACEY, J. I., and LACEY, B. C. (1958), 'Verification and extension of the principle of autonomic response stereotypy', *Amer. J. Psychol.*, vol. 71, pp. 50–73.

LACEY, J. I., and SMITH, R. I. (1954), 'Conditioning and generalization of unconscious anxiety', *Sci.*, vol. 120, pp. 1–8.

LADER, M. H. (1967), 'Palmar skin conductance measures in anxiety and phobic states', *J. psychosom. Res.*, vol. 11, pp. 271–81.

LADER, M. H., GELDER, M. G., and MARKS, I. M. (1967), 'Palmar skin conductance measures as predictors of response to desensitization', *J. psychosom. Res.*, vol. 11, pp. 283–90.

LADER, M. H., and MATHEWS, A. M. (1968), 'A physiological model of phobic anxiety and desensitization', *Behav. Res. Ther.*, vol. 6, pp. 411–21.

LADER, M. H., and WING, L. (1966), 'Physiological measures, sedative drugs and morbid anxiety', Oxford University Press.

LAING, R. D. (1960), *The Divided Self*, Tavistock.

LANDIS, C. A. (1937), 'Statistical evaluation of psychotherapeutic methods', in Hinsie, L. E. (ed.), *Concepts and Problems of Psychotherapy*, Columbia University Press.

LANG, P. J., and LAZOVIK, A. D. (1963), 'The experimental desensitization of phobia', *J. abnorm. soc. Psychol.*, vol. 66, pp. 519–25.

LANG, P. J., LAZOVIK, A. D., and REYNOLDS, D. J. (1966), 'Desensitization, suggestibility and pseudo-therapy', *J. abnorm. soc. Psychol.*, vol. 6, pp. 395–402.

LANYON, R. I., and MANOSEVITZ, M. (1966), 'Validity of self-reported fear', *Behav. Res. Ther.*, vol. 4, pp. 259–63.

LAURENCE, D. R. (1962), *Clinical Pharmacology*, Churchill.

LAZARUS, A. A. (1958), 'A new method in psychotherapy: a case study', *S. Afr. Med. J.*, vol. 33, pp. 660–63.

LAZARUS, A. A. (1959), 'The elimination of children's phobias by deconditioning', *Med. Proc. S. Afr.*, vol. 5, pp. 261–5.

LAZARUS, A. A. (1961a), 'Group therapy of phobic disorders by systematic desensitization', *J. abnorm. soc. Psychol.*, vol. 63, pp. 504–10.

LAZARUS, A. A. (1961b), 'Objective psychotherapy in treatment of dysphemia', *J. S. Afr. Logoped. Soc.*, pp. 8–10.

LAZARUS, A. A. (1963), 'The results of behaviour therapy in 126 cases of severe neurosis', *Behav. Res. Ther.*, vol. 1, pp. 69–79.

LAZARUS, A. A. (1964), 'Crucial procedural factors in desensitization therapy', *Behav. Res. Ther.*, vol. 2, pp. 65–70.

LAZARUS, A. A. (1966a), 'Behaviour rehearsal *v.* non-directive therapy *v.* advice in effecting behaviour change', *Behav. Res. Ther.*, vol. 4, pp. 209–12.

LAZARUS, A. A. (1966b), 'Broad spectrum behaviour therapy and the treatment of agoraphobia', *Behav. Res. Ther.*, vol. 4, pp. 95–7.

LAZARUS, A. A. (1968a), 'Learning theory and the treatment of depression', *Behav. Res. Ther.*, vol. 6, pp. 83–9.

LAZARUS, A. A. (1968b), 'Behaviour therapy and graded structure', in Porter, R. (ed.), *Symposium on the Role of Learning in Psychotherapy*, C.I.B.A. Foundation Symposium, Churchill.

LAZARUS, A. A. (1968c), *Behavior Therapy and Marriage Counseling*, unpublished manuscript, Eastern Pennsylvania Psychiatric Institute.

LAZARUS, A. A. (1968d), 'Variations in desensitization therapy', *Psychother.* vol. 5, pp. 50–52.

LAZARUS, A. A. (1968e), 'Behavior therapy in groups', in Gazda, C. M. (ed.), *Basic Approaches to Group Psychotherapy and Counseling*, Thomas.

LAZARUS, A. A., and ABRAMOVITZ, A. (1962), 'The use of "emotive imagery" in the treatment of children's phobias', *J. ment. Sci.*, vol. 108, pp. 131–5.

LAZARUS, A. A., DAVISON, G. C., and POLEFKA, D. A. (1965), 'Classical and operant factors in the treatment of a school phobia', *J. abnorm. soc. Psychol.*, vol. 70, pp. 225–9.

LAZARUS, A. A., and RACHMAN, S. (1960), 'The use of systematic desensitization in psychotherapy', in Eysenck, H. J. (ed.), *Behaviour Therapy and the Neuroses*, Pergamon Press.

LAZARUS, A. A., and SERBER, M. (1968), 'Is systematic desensitization being misapplied?', *Psychol. Rep.*, vol. 23, pp. 215–18.

LEFF, R. (1968), 'Behaviour modification and the psychoses of childhood: a review', *Psychol. Bull.*, vol. 69, pp. 396–409.

LEHNER, G. F. C. (1954), 'Negative practice as a psychotherapeutic technique', *J. Psychol.*, vol. 51, pp. 68–82.

LEITENBERG, H., AGRAS, W. S., BARLOW, D. H., and OLIVEAU, D. L. (1969), 'Contribution of selective positive reinforcement and therapeutic instructions to systematic desensitization therapy', *J. abnorm. Psychol.*, vol. 74, pp. 113–18.

LEMERE, F., and VOEGTLIN, W. L. (1950), 'An evaluation of the aversive treatment of alcoholism', *Q. J. Stud. Alcohol.*, vol. 11, pp. 199–204.

LEVINSON, F., and MEYER, V. (1965), 'Personality changes in relation to psychiatric status following orbital cortex undercutting', *Brit. J. Psychiat.*, vol. 111, pp. 207–18.

LEVIS, D. J., and CARRERA, R. N. (1967), 'Effects of ten hours of implosive therapy in the treatment of out-patients: a preliminary report', *J. abnorm. Psychol.*, vol. 72, pp. 504–8.

References

LEWIS, A. J. (1953), 'Health as a social concept', *Brit. J. Sociol.*, vol. 4, pp. 109–24.
LEWIS, A. J. (1957), 'Obsessional illness', *Alta Neuropsiquiat. Argent.*, vol. 3, pp. 323–34.
LEWIS, A. J. (1966), 'Psychological medicine', in Bodley Scott, R. (ed.), *Price's Textbook of Medicine*, Oxford University Press.
LIBERMAN, R. (1962), 'An analysis of the placebo phenomenon', *J. chron. Dis.*, vol. 15, pp. 761–83.
LIBERMAN, R. (1964), 'An experimental study of the placebo response under three different situations of pain', *J. psychiat. Res.*, vol. 2, pp. 233–46.
LIDDELL, H. S. (1944), 'Conditioned reflex method and experimental neurosis', in McV. Hunt, J. (ed.), *Personality and the Behavior Disorders*, Ronald Press.
LIDDELL, H. S. (1960), 'Experimental neuroses in animals', in Tanner, J. M. (ed.), *Stress and Psychiatric Disorder*, Blackwell.
LIDZ, T., FLECK, S., and CORNELISON, A. (1966), *Schizophrenia and the Family*, International Universities Press.
LINDSLEY, O. R. (1956), 'Operant conditioning methods applied to research in chronic schizophrenia', *Psychiat. Res. Rep.*, vol. 5 pp. 118–39.
LINDSLEY, O. R. (1960), 'Characteristics of the behavior of chronic psychotics as revealed by free-operant conditioning methods', *Dis. Nerv. Syst.*, Monograph Supplement, vol. 21, pp. 66–78.
LINDSLEY, O. R., and SKINNER, B. F. (1954), 'A method for the experimental analysis of the behavior of psychotic patients', *Amer. Psychol.*, vol. 9, pp. 419–20.
LIVERSEDGE, L. A., and SYLVESTER, J. D. (1955), 'Conditioning techniques in the treatment of writer's cramp', *Lancet*, vol. 1, pp. 1147–9.
LOMONT, J. F. (1965), 'Reciprocal inhibition or extinction?', *Behav. Res. Ther.*, vol. 3, pp. 209–19.
LOMONT, J. F., and EDWARDS, J. E. (1967), 'The role of relaxation in systematic desensitization', *Behav. Res. Ther.*, vol. 5, pp. 11–25.
LONDON, P. (1964), *The Modes and Morals of Psychotherapy*, Holt, Rinehart and Winston.
LOVAAS, O. I. (1961), 'Interaction between verbal and non-verbal behavior', *Child Develop.*, vol. 32, pp. 329–36.
LOVAAS, O. I. (1964), 'Clinical implications of the relationship between verbal and non-verbal operant behaviour', in Eysenck, H. J. (ed.), *Experiments in Behaviour Therapy*, Pergamon Press.
LOVAAS, O. I. (1966), 'A program for the establishment of speech in psychotic children', in Wing, J. K. (ed.), *Early Childhood Autism*, Pergamon Press.
LOVIBOND, S. H. (1964), *Conditioning and Enuresis*, Pergamon Press.
LUBORSKY, L., and STRUPP, H. H. (1962), 'Research problems in psychotherapy: a three-year follow-up', in Strupp, H. H., and Luborsky, L. (eds.), *Research in Psychotherapy*, vol. 2, A.P.A.

LUBY, E. D., and GOTTLIEB, E. D. (1968), 'Model psychoses', in Howells, J. G. (ed.), *Modern Perspectives in World Psychiatry*, Oliver and Boyd.

LURIA, A. R. (1961), *The Role of Speech in the Regulation of Normal and Abnormal Behaviour*, Pergamon Press.

MACCORQUODALE, K., and MEEHL, P. E. (1954), 'Edward C. Tolman', in Estes *et al.* (eds.), *Modern Learning Theory*, Appleton-Century-Crofts.

MACCULLOCH, M. J., and FELDMAN, M. P. (1967), 'Aversion therapy in management of forty-three homosexuals', *Brit. med. J.*, vol. 2, pp. 594–7.

MACCULLOCH, M. J., FELDMAN, M. P., and PINSHOFF, J. M. (1965), 'The application of anticipatory avoidance learning to the treatment of homosexuality. 2: Avoidance response latencies and pulse rate changes', *Behav. Res. Ther.*, vol. 3, pp. 21–43.

MACFARLANE, J. W., ALLEN, L., and HONZIK, M. (1954), *A Developmental Study of the Behavior Problems of Normal Children*, California University Press.

MCGUIRE, R. J., CARLISLE, J. M., and YOUNG, B. G. (1965), 'Sexual deviations as conditioned behaviour: a hypothesis', *Behav. Res. Ther.*, vol. 2, pp. 185–90.

MCGUIRE, R. L., and VALLANCE, M. (1964), 'Aversion therapy by electric shock: a simple technique', *Brit. med. J.*, vol. 1, pp. 151–3.

MACLAREN. J. (1960), 'The treatment of stammering by the Cherry–Sayers method: clinical impressions', in Eysenck, H. J. (ed.), *Behaviour Therapy and the Neuroses*, Pergamon Press.

MACPHERSON, E. L. R. (1967), 'Control of involuntary movement', *Behav. Res. Ther.*, vol. 5, pp. 143–5.

MADILL, M. F., CAMPBELL, D., LAVERTY, S. G., SANDERSON, R. E., and VANDERWATER S. L. (1966), 'Aversion treatment of alcoholics by succinylcholine-induced apnoeic paralysis', *Q. J. Stud. Alcohol.*, vol. 27, pp. 483–509.

MADSEN, C. H., and ULLMANN, L. P. (1967), 'Innovations in the desensitization of frigidity', *Behav. Res. Ther.*, vol. 5, pp. 67–8.

MAIER, N. (1949), *Frustration*, McGraw-Hill.

MAIER, N. (1956), 'Frustration theory', *Psychol. Rev.*, vol. 63, pp. 370–88.

MALAN, D. H., BACAL, H. A., HEATH, E. S., and BALFOUR, F. H. G. (1968), 'A study of psychodynamic changes in untreated neurotic patients', *Brit. J. Psychiat.*, vol. 114, pp. 525–51.

MALLESON, N. (1959), 'Panic and phobia', *Lancet*, vol. 1, pp. 225–7.

MALMO, R. B., DAVIS, J. F., and BARZA, S. (1952), 'Total hysterical deafness: an experimental study', *J. Person.*, vol. 21, pp. 188–204.

MALMO, R. B., and SHAGASS, C. (1949), 'Physiologic study of symptom mechanisms in psychiatric patients under stress', *Psychosom. Med.*, vol. 11, pp. 25–9.

MALMO, R. B., SHAGASS, C., and DAVIS, J. F. (1950), 'Symptom specificity and bodily reactions during psychiatric interview', *Psychosom. Med.*, vol. 12, pp. 362–76.

References

MANOSEVITZ, M., and LANYON, R. I. (1965), 'Fear survey schedule: a normative study', *Psychol. Rep.*, vol. 11, pp. 699–703.

MARKS, I. M. (1965), *Patterns of Meaning in Psychiatric Patients*, Maudsley Monographs, no. 13, Oxford University Press.

MARKS, I. M. (1968a), 'Aversion therapy', *Brit. J. med. Psychol.*, vol. 41, pp. 47–52.

MARKS, I. M. (1968b), personal communication to Meyer and Chesser.

MARKS, I. M., BIRLEY, J., and GELDER M. G. (1966), 'Modified leucotomy in severe agoraphobia: a controlled serial inquiry', *Brit. J. Psychiat.*, vol. 112, pp. 757–69.

MARKS, I. M., and GELDER, M. G. (1965), 'A controlled retrospective study of behaviour therapy in phobic patients', *Brit. J. Psychiat.*, vol. 111, pp. 561–73.

MARKS, I. M., and GELDER, M. G. (1966), 'Common ground between behaviour therapy and psychodynamic methods', *Brit. J. med. Psychol.*, vol. 39, pp. 11–23.

MARKS, I. M., and GELDER M. G. (1967), 'Transvestism and fetishism: clinical and psychological changes during faradic aversion', *Brit. J. Psychiat.*, vol. 113, pp. 711–29.

MARKS, I. M., GELDER, M. G., and EDWARDS, G. (1968), 'Hypnosis and desensitization for phobias: a controlled prospective trial', *Brit. J. Psychiat.*, vol. 114, pp. 1263–74.

MARKS, I. M., and SARTORIUS, N. H. (1968), 'A contribution to the measurement of sexual attitude', *J. nerv. ment. Dis.*, vol. 145, pp. 441–51.

MARLAND, P. M. (1956), 'Notes on some preliminary clinical trials: appendix to experiments upon the total inhibition of stammering by external control – Cherry, C., and Sayers, B.McA.', *J. psychosom. Res.*, vol. 1, pp. 233–46.

MARTIN, B. (1961), 'The assessment of anxiety by physiological behaviour measures', *Psychol. Bull.*, vol. 58, pp. 234–55. .

MARTIN, B. (1969), 'Anxiety', in Costello, C. G. (ed.), *Symptoms of Psychopathology*, Wiley.

MARTIN, I. (1960), 'Somatic reactivity', in Eysenck, H. J. (ed.), *Handbook of Abnormal Psychology*, Pitman.

MARTIN, I. (1964), 'Adaptation', *Psychol. Bull.*, vol. 61, pp. 35–44.

MARTIN, I., MARKS, I. M., and GELDER, M. G. (1969), 'Conditioned eyelid responses in phobic patients', *Behav. Res. Ther.*, vol. 7, pp. 115–24.

MARTIN, G. L., ENGLAND, G., KAPRANY, E., KILGOUR, K., and PILEK, V. (1968), 'Operant conditioning of kindergarten-class behaviour in autistic children', *Behav. Res. Ther.*, vol. 6, pp. 281–94.

MASON, J. W., BRADY, J. V., and TOLSON, W. W. (1966), 'Behavioural adaptations and endocrine activity', *Res. Publ. Ass. nerv. ment. Dis.*, vol. 43, pp. 227–50.

MASSERMAN, J. H. (1964), *Behavior and Neurosis*, Hafner.

MAX, L. W. (1935), 'Breaking up a homosexual fixation by the conditioned reaction technique: a case study', *Psychol. Bull.*, vol. 32, pp. 734.

MAY, R. (1950), *The Meaning of Anxiety*, Ronald Press.

MEEHL, P. E. (1950), 'On the circularity of the law of effect', *Psychol. Bull.*, vol. 47, pp. 52–75.

MEISSNER, J. H. (1946), 'The relationship between voluntary non-fluency and stuttering', *J. Speech Disord.*, vol. 11, pp. 13–33.

METCALFE, M. (1956), 'Demonstration of psychosomatic relationships', *Brit. J. med. Psychol.*, vol. 29, pp. 63–6.

METZNER, R. (1961), 'Learning theory and the therapy of neurosis', *Brit. J. Psychol.*, Monog. Suppl., no. 33.

METZNER, R. (1963), 'Some experimental analogues of obsession', *Behav. Res. Ther.*, vol. 1, pp. 231–6.

MEYER, V. (1957), 'The treatment of two phobic patients on the basis of learning principles', *J. abnorm. soc. Psychol.*, vol. 55, pp. 261–6.

MEYER, V. (1966), 'Modification of expectations in cases with obsessional rituals', *Behav. Res. Ther.*, vol. 4, pp. 273–80.

MEYER, V., and CRISP, A. H. (1964), 'Aversion therapy in two cases of obesity', *Behav. Res. Ther.*, vol. 2, pp. 143–7.

MEYER, V., and CRISP, A. H. (1966), 'Some problems in behaviour therapy', *Brit. J. Psychiat.*, vol. 112, pp. 367–81.

MEYER, V., and GELDER, M. G. (1963), 'Behaviour therapy and phobic disorders', *Brit. J. Psychiat.*, vol. 109, pp. 19–28.

MEYER, V., and MAIR, J. M. M. (1963), 'A new technique to control stammering: a preliminary report', *Behav. Res. Ther.*, vol. 1, pp. 251–4.

MICHENBAUM, D. H. (1966), 'The effects of social reinforcement on the level of abstraction in schizophrenics', *J. abnorm. Psychol.*, vol. 71, pp. 354–63.

MIGLER, B., and WOLPE, J. (1967), 'Automated self-desensitization: a case report', *Behav. Res. Ther.*, vol. 5, pp. 133–5.

MILLER, N. E. (1944), 'Experimental studies of conflict', in Hunt, J. McV. (ed.), *Personality and the Behavior Disorders*, Ronald Press.

MILLER, N. E. (1948), 'Studies of fear as an acquired drive', *J. exp. Psychol.*, vol. 38, pp. 89–101.

MILLER, N. E., and DOLLARD, J. C. (1941), *Social Learning and Imitation*, Yale University Press.

MILLER, R. E., BANKS, J. H., and OGAWA, N. (1962), 'Communication of affect in "co-operation conditioning" of rhesus monkeys', *J. abnorm. soc. Pyschol.*, vol. 64, pp. 343–8.

MILLER, R. E., BANKS, J. H., and OGAWA, N. (1963), 'Role of facial expression in "co-operative avoidance conditioning" in monkeys', *J. abnorm. soc. Psychol.*, vol. 67, pp. 24–30.

MOORE, N. (1965), 'Behaviour therapy in bronchial asthma: a controlled study', *J. psychosom. Res.*, vol. 9, pp. 257–76.

263

References

MORGENSTERN, F. S., PEARCE, J. F., and REES, L. W. (1965), 'Predicting outcome of behaviour therapy by psychological tests', *Behav. Res. Ther.*, vol. 2, pp. 191–200.

MOWRER, O. H. (1947), 'On the dual nature of learning – a reinterpretation of "conditioning" and "problem solving"', *Harvard educ. Rev.*, vol. 17., pp. 102–48.

MOWRER, O. H. (1950), *Learning Theory and Personality Dynamics*, Ronald Press.

MOWRER, O. H. (1960), *Learning Theory and Behavior*, Wiley.

MOWRER, O. H., and MOWRER, W. M. (1938), 'Enuresis: a method for its study and treatment', *Amer. J. Orthopsychiat.*, vol. 8, pp. 436–59.

MOWRER, O. H., and VIEK, P. (1948), 'An experimental analogue of fear from a sense of helplessness', *J. abnorm. soc. Psychol.*, vol. 67, pp. 24–30.

MURPHY, J. V., MILLER, R. E., and MIRSKY, I. A. (1955), 'Inter-animal conditioning in the monkey', *J. comp. physiol. Psychol.*, vol. 48, pp. 211–14.

NAGEL, E. (1959), 'Methodological issues in psychoanalytical theory', in Hook, S. (ed.), *Psychoanalysis, Scientific Method and Philosophy*, New York University Press.

NAPALKOV, A. V. (1963), 'Information process of the brain', in Wiener, N., and Schade, J. P. (eds.), *Progress in Brain Research*, vol. 2, *Nerve, Brain and Memory Models*, Elsevier Publishing Co.

NEAL, D. H. (1963), 'Behaviour therapy and encopresis in children', *Behav. Res. Ther.*, vol. 1, pp. 139–49.

O'CONNOR, N., and FRANKS, C. (1960), 'Childhood upbringing and other environmental factors', in Eysenck, H. J. (ed.), *Handbook of Abnormal Psychology*, Pitman.

OLDS, J. (1963), 'Mechanisms of instrumental conditioning', *Electroenceph. clin. Neurophysiol. Suppl.*, vol. 24, pp. 219–34.

O'LEARY, K. D., O'LEARY, S., and BECKER, W. C. (1967), 'Modification of a deviant sibling interaction pattern in the home', *Behav. Res. Ther.*, vol. 5, pp. 113–20.

OLIVEAU, D. L., AGRAS, W. S., LEITENBERG, H., MOORE, R. C., and WRIGHT, D. E. (1969), 'Systematic desensitization, therapeutically oriented instructions and selective positive reinforcement', *Behav. Res. Ther.*, vol. 7, pp. 27–33.

O'NEILL, D. G., and HOWELL, R. J. (1969), 'Three modes of hierarchy presentation in systematic desensitization therapy', *Behav. Res. Ther.*, vol. 7, pp. 289–94.

OSGOOD, C. E. (1953), *Method and Theory in Experimental Psychology*, Oxford University Press.

PARK, L. C., and COVI, L. (1965), 'Non-blind placebo trial', *Arch. gen. Psychiat.*, vol. 12, pp. 536–45.

PATTERSON, G. R. (1965), 'A learning theory approach to the treatment of the school phobic child', in Ullmann, L. P., and Krasner, L. (eds.), *Case Studies in Behavior Modification*, Holt, Rinehart and Winston.

PATTERSON, G. R., JONES, R., WHITTIER, J., and WRIGHT, M. A. (1965), 'A behaviour modification technique for the hyperactive child', *Behav. Res. Ther.*, vol. 2, pp. 217–26.

PAUL, G. L. (1966), *Insight v. Desensitization in Psychotherapy: An Experiment in Anxiety Reduction*, Stanford University Press.

PAUL, G. L. (1967), 'Insight versus desensitization in psychotherapy two years after termination', *J. cons. Psychol.*, vol. 31, pp. 333–48.

PAUL, G. L. (1968), 'Two-year follow-up of systematic desensitization in a therapy group', *J. abnorm. Psychol.*, vol. 73, pp. 119–30.

PAUL, G. L., and SHANNON, D. T. (1966), 'Treatment of anxiety through systematic desensitization in therapy groups', *J. abnorm. soc. Psychol.*, vol. 71, pp. 124–35.

PAVLOV, I. P. (1927), *Conditioned Reflexes*, Oxford University Press.

PETERS, H. N., and JENKINS, R. L. (1954), 'Improvement of chronic schizophrenic patients with guided problem solving motivated by hunger', *Psychiat. Q. Suppl.*, vol. 28, pp. 84–101.

PETERSON, D. R., and LONDON, P. (1965), 'A role for cognition in the behavioral treatment of a child's eliminative disturbance', in Ullmann, L. P., and Krasner, L. (eds.), *Case Studies in Behavior Modification*, Holt, Rinehart and Winston.

PHILLIPS, E. L., and WIENER, D. N. (1966), *Short-Term Psychotherapy and Structural Behavior Change*, McGraw-Hill.

PIERS, G., and PIERS, M. W. (1965), 'Modes of learning and the analytic process', *Proc. 6th Int. Cong. Psychother.*, vol. 4, pp. 104–10.

POLIN, A. T. (1959), 'The effect of flooding and physical suppression as extinction techniques on an anxiety-motivated avoidance locomotor response', *J. Psychol.*, vol. 47, pp. 253–5.

POLLIT, J. (1960), 'Natural history studies in mental illness: a discussion based on a pilot study of obsessional states', *J. ment. Sci.*, vol. 106, pp. 93–113.

POPOVIC, M., and PETROVIC, D. (1964), 'After the earthquake', *Lancet*, vol. 2, pp. 1169–71.

POPPER, K. R. (1963), 'Science: conjectures and refutations', in *Conjectures and Refutations*, Routledge and Kegan Paul.

POSER, E. G. (1967), 'Training behaviour therapists', *Behav. Res. Ther.*, vol. 5, pp. 37–41.

PREMACK, D. (1959), 'Towards empirical behaviour laws. 1: Positive reinforcement', *Psychol. Rev.*, vol. 66, pp. 219–33.

PRIBRAM, K. H. (1961), 'Implications for systematic studies of behavior', in Sheer, D. E. (ed.), *Electrical Stimulation of the Brain*, Texas University Press.

References

PRIBRAM, K. H. (1963), 'A neuropsychological model', in Knapp, P. H. (ed.), *Expressions of the Emotions in Man*, International Universities Press.

RACHMAN, S. (1957), personal communication, quoted in Wolpe, J. (1958), *Psychotherapy by Reciprocal Inhibition*, Stanford University Press.

RACHMAN, S. (1963), 'Spontaneous remission and latent learning', *Behav. Res. Ther.*, vol. 1, pp. 133–7.

RACHMAN, S. (1965a), 'Aversion therapy: chemical or electrical', *Behav. Res. Ther.*, vol. 2, pp. 289–99.

RACHMAN, S. (1965b), 'Studies in desensitization. 1: The separate effects of relaxation and desensitization', *Behav. Res. Ther.*, vol. 3, pp. 245–51.

RACHMAN, S. (1966a), 'Studies in desensitization. 2: Flooding', *Behav. Res. Ther.*, vol. 4, pp. 1–6.

RACHMAN, S. (1966b), 'Studies in desensitization. 3: Speed of generalization', *Behav. Res. Ther.*, vol. 4, pp. 7–15.

RACHMAN, S. (1966c), 'Sexual fetishism: an experimental analogue', *Psychol. Rec.*, vol. 16, pp. 293–6.

RACHMAN, S. (1968), 'The role of muscular relaxation in desensitization therapy', *Behav. Res. Ther.*, vol. 6, pp. 159–66.

RACHMAN, S., and EYSENCK, H. J. (1966), 'Reply to a "critique and reformulation" of behavior therapy', *Psychol. Bull.*, vol. 65, pp. 165–9.

RACHMAN, S., and HODGSON, R. J. (1967), 'Studies in desensitization. 4: Optimum degree of anxiety-reduction', *Behav. Res. Ther.*, vol. 5, pp. 249–50.

RAFI, A. A. (1962), 'Learning theory and the treatment of tics', *J. psychosom. Res.*, vol. 6, pp. 71–6.

RAMSAY, R. W., BARENDS, J., BRUCHER, J., and KRUSEMAN, A. (1966), 'Massed versus spaced desensitization of fear', *Behav. Res. Ther.*, vol. 4, pp. 205–7.

RAPAPORT, D. (1960), 'The structure of psychoanalytical theory', *Psychol. Iss.*, vol. 2, no. 2.

RAYMOND, M. J. (1964), 'The treatment of addiction by aversion conditioning with apomorphine', *Behav. Res. Ther.*, vol. 1, pp. 287–91.

RAZRAN, G. (1939), 'A quantitative study of meaning by a conditioned salivary technique (semantic conditioning)', *Science*, vol. 90, pp. 89–91.

RAZRAN, G. (1965), 'Russian psychologists' psychology and American experimental psychology', *Psychol. Bull.*, vol. 63, pp. 42–64.

REED, J. L. (1966), 'Comments on the use of methohexitone sodium as a means of inducing relaxation', *Behav. Res. Ther.*, vol. 4, p. 323.

RICE, D. G. (1966), 'Operant conditioning and associated electromyogram responses', *J. exp. Psychol.*, vol. 71, pp. 908–12.

RIMLAND, B. (1964), *Infantile Autism*, Appleton-Century-Crofts.

RISLEY, T., and WOLF, M. (1967), 'Establishing functional speech in echolalic children', *Behav. Res. Ther.*, vol. 5, pp. 73–88.

RITTER, B. (1968), 'The group desensitization of children's snake phobias using vicarious and contact desensitization procedures', *Behav. Res. Ther.*, vol. 6, pp. 1–6.

ROGERS, C. R. (1951), *Client-Centred Therapy*, Houghton Mifflin.

ROSENBERG, C. M. (1967), 'Personality and obsessional neurosis', *Brit. J. Psychiat.*, vol .113, pp. 471–7.

ROSENTHAL, R. (1966), *Experimenter Effects in Behavioral Research*, Appleton-Century-Crofts.

RUBIN, B. M., KATKIN, E. W., WEISS, B. W., and EFRAN, J. S. (1968), 'Factor analysis of a fear survey schedule', *Behav. Res. Ther.*, vol. 6, pp. 65–75.

RUSSO, S. (1964), 'Adaptations in behavioural therapy with children', *Behav. Res. Ther.*, vol. 2, pp. 43–7.

RYCROFT, C. (1966), 'Causes and meaning', in Rycroft, C. (ed.), *Psychoanalysis Observed*, Constable.

SACHS, E. (1967), 'Dissociation of learning in rats and its similarities to dissociative states in man', in Zubin, J., and Hunt, H. F. (eds.), *Comparative Psychopathology*, Grune and Stratton.

SANDERSON, R. E., CAMPBELL, D., and LAVERTY, S. (1963), 'Traumatically conditioned responses acquired during respiratory paralysis', *Nature*, vol. 196, pp. 1235–6.

SANDERSON, R., CAMPBELL, D., and LAVERTY, S. (1964), 'An investigation of a new aversive conditioning technique for alcoholism', in Franks, C. M. (ed.), *Conditioning Techniques in Clinical Practice and Research*, Springer.

SARGANT, W., (1957), *Battle for the Mind*, Heinemann.

SAWREY, W. L., CONGER, J. J., and TURRELL, E. S. (1956), 'Experimental investigation of the role of psychological factors in production of gastric ulcers in rats', *J. comp. physiol. Psychol.*, vol. 49, pp. 457–61.

SCHACHTER, S. (1964), 'The interaction of cognitive and physiological determinants of emotional state', in Berkowitz, L. (ed.), *Advances in Experimental Social Psychology*, vol. 1, Academic Press.

SCHEFLEN, N. A. (1957), 'Generalization and extinction of experimentally induced fears in cats', in Hoch, P. H., and Zubin, J. (eds.), *Experimental Psychopathology*, Grune and Stratton.

SCHLOSBERG, H. (1937), 'The relationship between success and the laws of conditioning', *Psychol. Rev.*, vol. 44, pp. 379–94.

SCHMIDT, E., CASTELL, D., and BROWN, P. (1965), 'A retrospective study of forty-two cases of behaviour therapy', *Behav. Res. Ther.*, vol. 3, pp. 9–19.

SCHULTZ, J. H., and LUTHE, W. (1959), *Autogenic Training: A Psychophysiological Approach to Psychotheraphy*, Grune and Stratton.

SCHWITZGEBEL, R., and KOLB, D. A. (1964), 'Inducing behaviour change in adolescent delinquents', *Behav. Res. Ther.*, vol. 1, pp. 297–304.

SENAY, E. C. (1966), 'Towards an animal model of depression: a study of separation behaviour in dogs', *J. psychiat. Res.*, vol. 4, pp. 65–71.

References

SERGEANT, H. G. S., and YORKSTON, N. J. (1968), 'Some complications of using methohexitone to relax anxious patients', *Lancet*, vol. 2, pp. 653–5.

SHAND, A. F. (1914), *The Foundations of Character*, Macmillan.

SHAPIRO, A. K. (1968), 'The placebo response', in Howells, J. G. (ed.), *Modern Perspective in World Psychiatry*, Oliver and Boyd.

SHEEHAN, J. G. (1951), 'The modification of stuttering through non-reinforcement', *J. abnorm. soc. Psychol.*, vol. 46, pp. 51–63.

SHEEHAN, J. G., and VOAS, R. B. (1957), 'Stuttering as conflict. 1: Comparison of therapy techniques involving approach and avoidance', *J. Speech Dis.*, vol. 22, pp. 714–23.

SHEPHERD, M., COOPER, B., BROWN, A. C., and KALTON, G. W. (1966), *Psychiatric Illness in General Practice*, Oxford University Press.

SHERMAN, J. A. (1965), 'Use of reinforcement and imitation to reinstate verbal behaviour in mute psychotics', *J. abnorm. soc. Psychol.*, vol. 70, pp. 155–64.

SHOBEN, E. J. (1949), 'Psychotherapy as a problem in learning theory', *Psychol. Bull.*, vol. 46, pp. 366–92.

SIDMAN, M. (1962), 'Operant techniques', in Bachrach, A. (ed.), *Experimental Foundation of Clinical Psychology*, Basic Books.

SIDMAN, M., HERRENSTEIN, R. J., and CONRAD, D. G. (1957), 'Maintenance of avoidance behavior by unavoidable shocks', *J. comp. physiol. Psychol.*, vol. 50, pp. 553–7.

SINGER, M. T., and WYNNE, L. C. (1965), 'Thought disorder and family relations of schizophrenics. 4: Results and implications', *Arch. gen. Psychiat.*, vol. 12, pp. 201–12.

SKINNER, B. F. (1938), *The Behavior of Organisms*, Appleton-Century-Crofts.

SKINNER, B. F. (1948), 'Superstition in the pigeon', *J. exp. Psychol.*, vol. 38, pp. 168–72.

SKINNER, B. F. (1953), *Science and Human Behavior*, Macmillan Co.

SNAITH, R. P. (1968), 'A clinical investigation of phobia', *Brit. J. Psychiat.*, vol. 114, pp. 673–97.

SOKOLOV, Y. N., (1963), *Perception and the Conditioned Reflex*, Pergamon Press.

SOLOMON, R. L. (1964), 'Punishment', *Amer. Psychol.*, vol. 19, pp. 239–53.

SOLOMON, R. L. (1967), 'Aversive control in relation to the development of behavior disorders', in Zubin, J., and Hunt, R. F. (eds.), *Comparative Psychopathology*, Grune and Stratton.

SOLOMON, R. L., and WYNNE, L. C. (1953), 'Traumatic avoidance learning: acquisition in normal dogs', *Psychol. Monogr.*, vol. 67, no. 4, whole no. 354.

SOLOMON, R. L., and WYNNE, L. C. (1954), 'Traumatic avoidance learning: the principle of anxiety conservation and partial irreversibility', *Psychol. Rev.*, vol. 81, pp. 353–85.

SOLYOM, L., and MILLER, S. B. (1967), 'Reciprocal inhibition by aversion relief in the treatment of phobias', *Behav. Res. Ther.*, vol. 5, pp. 313–24.

268

SPENCE, K. W. (1964), 'Anxiety (drive) level and performance in eyelid conditioning', *Psychol. Bull.*, vol. 61, pp. 129–39.

STAATS, A. W., and STAATS, C. K. (1963), *Complex Human Behavior: A Systematic Extension of Learning Principles*, Holt, Rinehart and Winston.

STAATS, A. W., MINKE, K. A., GOODWIN, W., and LANDEEN, J. (1967), 'Cognitive behaviour modification: "motivated learning" reading treatment with sub-professional therapy-technicians', *Behav. Res. Ther.*, vol. 5, pp. 283–99.

STAFFORD-CLARK, D. (1963), *Psychiatry for Students*, Allen and Unwin.

STAMPFL, T. G., and LEVIS, D. J. (1967), 'The essentials of implosive therapy: a learning-theory-based psychodynamic behavioural therapy', *J. abnorm. soc. Psychol.*, vol. 72, pp. 496–503.

STAMPFL, T. G., and LEVIS, D. J. (1968), 'Implosive therapy – a behavioural therapy?' *Behav. Res. Ther.*, vol. 6, pp. 31–6.

STAUB, E. (1968), 'Duration of stimulus exposure as determinant of the efficacy of flooding procedures in the elimination of fears', *Behav. Res. Ther.*, vol. 6, pp. 131–2.

STEIN, L. (1966), 'Habituation and stimulus novelty: a model based on classical conditioning', *Psychol. Rev.*, vol. 73, pp. 352–6.

STENGEL, E. (1959), 'Classification of mental disorders', *W.H.O. Bull.*, vol. 21, pp. 601–63.

STEPHENS, J. H., and GANTT, W. H. (1956), 'The differential effects of morphine on cardiac and motor conditioned reflexes', *Bull. Johns Hopkins Hospital*, vol. 98, pp. 245–54.

STORR, A. (1966), 'The concept of cure', in Rycroft, C. (ed.), *Psychoanalysis Observed*, Constable.

STRAUGHAM, J. (1964), 'Treatment with child and mother in the playroom', *Behav. Res. Ther.*, vol. 2, pp. 37–41.

STRUPP, H. H., and BERGIN, A. E. (1969), 'Some empirical and conceptual bases for coordinated research in psychotherapy', *Int. J. Psychiat.*, vol. 7, pp. 18–168.

SULLIVAN, H. S. (1953), *The Interpersonal Theory of Psychiatry*, Norton.

SULLIVAN, H. S. (1955), *Conceptions of Modern Psychiatry*, Tavistock.

SYLVESTER, J. D., and LIVERSEDGE, L. A. (1960), 'Conditioning and the occupational cramp', in Eysenck, H. J. (ed.), *Behaviour Therapy and the Neuroses*, Pergamon Press.

SZASZ, T. S. (1961), *The Myth of Mental Illness*, Hoeber.

TAYLOR, F. K. (1966), *Psychopathology: Its Causes and Symptoms*, Butterworth.

TAYLOR, J. A. (1953), 'A personality scale of manifest anxiety', *J. abnorm. soc. Psychol.*, vol. 48, pp. 285–90.

THIMANN, J. (1949), 'Conditioned reflex treatment of alcoholism. 2: The risk of its application, its indications, contra-indications and psychotherapeutic methods', *New Eng. J. Med.*, vol. 241, pp. 408–10.

References

THOMPSON, R. F., and SPENCER, W. A. (1966), 'Habituation: a model phenomenon for the study of neuronal substrates of behavior', *Psychol. Rev.*, vol. 73, pp. 16–43.

THORNDIKE, E. L. (1911), *Animal Intelligence*, Macmillan Co.

THORPE, J. G., and SCHMIDT, E. (1964), 'Therapeutic failure in a case of aversion therapy', *Behav. Res. Ther.*, vol. 1, pp. 293–6.

THORPE, J. G., SCHMIDT, E., and CASTELL, D. (1964a), 'A comparison of positive and negative (aversive) conditioning in the treatment of homosexuality', *Behav. Res. Ther.*, vol. 1, pp. 357–62.

THORPE, J., SCHMIDT, E., BROWN, P. Y., and CASTELL, D. (1964b), 'Aversion relief therapy: a new method for general application', *Behav. Res. Ther.*, vol. 2, pp. 71–82.

TOLMAN, E. C. (1932), *Purposive Behavior in Animal and Men*, Appleton-Century-Crofts.

TRUAX, C. B. (1966a), 'Therapist empathy, warmth and genuineness and patient personality change in group psychotherapy: a comparison between interaction unit measures, time sample measures, patient perception measures', *J. clin. Psychol.*, vol. 22, pp. 225–9.

TRUAX, C. B. (1966b), 'Reinforcement and non-reinforcement in Rogerian psychotherapy', *J. abnorm. soc. Psychol.*, vol. 71, pp. 1–9.

TRUAX, C. B., and CARKHUFF, R. R. (1963), 'For better or for worse: the process of psychotherapeutic personality change', in *Recent Advances in the Study of Behavioral Change*, McGill University Press.

TRUAX, C. B., and CARKHUFF, R. R. (1964), 'Significant developments in psychotherapy research', in Abt, L. E., and Reiss, B. F. (eds.), *Progress in Clinical Psychology*, Grune and Stratton.

TRUAX, R. B., FINE, H., MORAVEC, J., and MILLIS, W. (1968), 'Effects of therapist persuasive potency in individual psychotherapy', *J. clin. Psychol.*, vol. 24, pp. 359–62.

TURNBULL, J. W. (1962), 'Asthma conceived as a learned response', *J. psychosom. Res.*, vol. 6, pp. 59–70.

TURNER, L. H., and SOLOMON, R. L. (1962), 'Human traumatic avoidance learning: theory and experiments on the operant–respondent distinction and failure to learn', *Psychol. Monogr.*, no. 76, whole no. 559.

TURNER, R. K., and YOUNG, G. C. (1966), 'C.N.S. stimulant drugs and conditioning treatment of nocturnal enuresis: a long term follow-up study', *Behav. Res. Ther.*, vol. 4, pp. 225–8.

TYHURST, J. S. (1951), 'Individual reactions to community disaster: the natural history of psychiatric phenomena', *Amer. J. Psychiat.*, vol. 107, pp. 764–9.

UHLENHUTH, E. H., CANTER, A., NEUXTADT, J. O., and PAYSON, H. E., (1959), 'The symptomatic relief of anxiety with meprobamate, phenobarbital and placebo', *Amer. J. Psychiat.*, vol. 115, pp. 905–10.

ULLMANN, L. P., FORSMAN, R. G., KENNY, J. W., MCINNIS, T. L., UNIKEL, I. P., and ZEISETT, R. M. (1965), 'Selective reinforcement of schizophrenics' interview responses', *Behav. Res. Ther.*, vol. 2, pp. 205–12.

ULLMANN, L. P., and KRASNER, L. (eds.) (1965), *Case Studies in Behavior Modification*, Holt, Rhinehart and Winston.

ULLMANN, L. P., KRASNER, L., and COLLINS, B. (1961a), 'Modification of behavior in group therapy associated with verbal conditioning', *J. abnorm. soc. Psychol.*, vol. 62, pp. 128–32.

ULLMANN, L. P., KRASNER, L., and EKMAN, P. (1961b), 'Verbal conditioning of emotional words: effects of behavior on group therapy', *Research Reports of VA Palo Alto*, no. 15.

ULLMANN, L. P., KRASNER, L., and EDINGER, R. L. (1964), 'Verbal conditioning of common associations in long-term schizophrenic patients', *Behav. Res. Ther.*, vol. 2, pp. 15–18.

VALINS, S., and RAY, A. A. (1967), 'Effect of cognitive desensitization on avoidance behaviour', *J. Personal. soc. Psychol.*, vol. 7, pp. 345–50.

VALLANCE, M. (1965), 'Alcoholism: a two year follow-up study', *Brit. J. Psychiat.*, vol. 111, pp. 348–56.

VENABLES, P. H., and MARTIN, I. (eds.) (1967), *A Manual of Psychophysiological Methods*, North-Holland Publishing Co.

WALLERSTEIN, R. S. (1957), *Hospital Treatment of Alcoholism: A Comparative Experimental Study*, Basic Books.

WALTON, D. (1960), 'The application of learning theory to the treatment of a case of neuro-dermatitis', in Eysenck, H. J. (ed.), *Behaviour Therapy and the Neuroses*, Pergamon Press.

WALTON, D. (1961), 'Experimental psychology and the treatment of a tiqueur', *J. child Psychol.*, vol. 2, pp. 148–55.

WALTON, D. (1964), 'Massed practice and simultaneous reduction in drive level – further evidence of the efficacy of this approach to the treatment of tics', in Eysenck, J. H. (ed.), *Experiments in Behaviour Therapy*, Pergamon Press.

WALTON, D., and MATHER, M. D. (1963), 'The application of learning principles to the treatment of obsessive-compulsive states in the acute and chronic phases of illness', *Behav. Res. Ther.*, vol. 1, pp. 163–74.

WATSON, J. B., and RAYNER, R. (1920), 'Conditioned emotional reactions', *J. exp. Psychol.*, vol. 3, pp. 1–14.

WERRY, J. S., and COHRSSEN, J. (1965), 'Enuresis – an etiologic and therapeutic study', *J. Pediat.*, vol. 67, pp. 423–31.

WHALER, G. R., WINKEL, G. H., PETERSON, R. F., and MORRISON, D. C. (1965), 'Mothers as behaviour therapists for their own children', *Behav. Res. Ther.*, vol. 3, pp. 113–24.

W.H.O. (1962), 'Deprivation of maternal care', *Public Health Papers*, no. 14, World Health Organization.

References

WIKLER, A. (1968), 'Interaction of physical dependence and classical and operant conditioning in the genesis of relapse', *Res. Publ. Ass. nerv. ment. Dis.*, no. 46, pp. 280–87.

WILDE, G. J. S. (1964), 'Behaviour therapy for addicted cigarette smokers: a preliminary investigation', *Behav. Res. Ther.*, vol. 2, pp. 107–9.

WILLIAMS, J. H. (1964), 'Conditioning of verbalization', *Psychol. Bull.*, vol. 62, pp. 383–93.

WILSON, G. D. (1967), 'Efficacy of "flooding" procedures in desensitization of fear: a theoretical note', *Behav. Res. Ther.*, vol. 5, p. 138.

WILSON, G. T., and DAVISON, G. C. (1969), 'Aversion techniques in behavior therapy: some theoretical and meta-theoretical considerations', *J. cons. Psychol.*, vol. 33, pp. 237–9.

WILSON, G. T., and EVANS, W. I. M. (1967), 'Behaviour therapy and not behaviour therapies', *Newsletter*, Assoc. Advance Behav. Ther., vol. 2, no. 3, pp. 5–7.

WILSON, G. T., HANNON, A. E., and EVANS, W. I. M. (1968), 'Behaviour therapy and the therapist–patient relationship', *J. cons. Psychol.*, vol. 32, pp. 103–9.

WILSON, A., and SMITH, F. J. (1968), 'Counter-conditioning therapy using free associations: pilot study', *J. abnorm. Psychol.*, vol. 73, pp. 474–8.

WILSON, F. S., and WALTERS, R. H. (1966), 'Modification of speech output of near-mute schizophrenics through social learning procedures', *Behav. Res. Ther.*, vol. 4, pp. 59–67.

WOLF, M., RISLEY, T., and MEES, H. (1964), 'Application of operant conditioning procedures to the behaviour problems of an autistic child', *Behav. Res. Ther.* vol. 1, pp. 305–12.

WOLPE, J. (1952), 'Experimental neuroses as learned behaviour', *Brit. J. Psychol.*, vol. 43, pp. 243–68.

WOLPE, J. (1958), *Psychotherapy by Reciprocal Inhibition*, Stanford University Press.

WOLFE, J. (1961), 'The systematic desensitization treatment of neuroses', *J. nerv. ment. Dis.*, vol. 132, pp. 189–203.

WOLPE, J. (1963), 'Quantitative relationships in the systematic desensitization of phobias', *Amer. J. Psychiat.*, vol. 119, pp. 1062–8.

WOLPE, J., and LANG, P. J. (1964), 'A fear schedule for use in behaviour therapy', *Behav. Res. Ther.*, vol. 2, pp. 27–30.

WOLPE, J., and LAZARUS, A. (1966), *Behaviour Therapy Techniques*, Pergamon Press.

WOLPIN, M., and RAINES, J. (1966), 'Visual imagery, expected roles and extinction as possible factors in reducing fear and avoidance behaviour', *Behav. Res. Ther.*, vol. 4, pp. 25–37.

WORSLEY, J. L., and FREEMAN, H. (1967), 'Further comments on the use of methohexitone sodium as a means of inducing relaxation', *Behav. Res. Ther.*, vol. 5, p. 258.

References

YATES, A. J. (1958), 'The application of learning theory to the treatment of tics', *J. abnorm. soc. Psychol.*, vol. 56, pp. 175–82.

YATES, A. J. (1962), *Frustration and Conflict*, Methuen.

YATES, A. J. (1963), 'Recent empirical and theoretical approaches to the experimental manipulation of speech in normal subjects and stammerers', *Behav. Res. Ther.*, vol. 1, pp. 95–119.

YEUNG, D. P. H. (1968), 'Diazepam for treatment of phobias', *Lancet*, vol. 1, pp. 475–6.

YORKSTON, N. J., SERGEANT, H. G. S., and RACHMAN, S. (1968), 'Methohexitone relaxation for desensitizing agoraphobic patients', *Lancet*, vol 2, pp. 651–3.

YOUNG, G. C. (1965), 'Personality factors and the treatment of enuresis', *Behav. Res. Ther.*, vol. 3, pp. 103–105.

YOUNG, G. C., and TURNER, R. K. (1965), 'C.N.S. stimulant drugs and conditioning treatment of nocturnal enuresis', *Behav. Res. Ther.*, vol. 3, pp. 93–101.

ZAX, M., and KLEIN, A. (1960), 'Measurement of personality and behavior changes following psychotherapy', *Psychol. Bull.*, vol. 57, pp. 435–48.

ZEISSET, R. M. (1968), 'Desensitization and relaxation in the modification of psychiatric patients' interview behavior', *J. abnorm. soc. Psychol.*, vol. 73, pp. 18–24.

ZIMMERMAN, J., and GROSZ, H. J. (1966), ' "Visual" performance of a functionally blind person', *Behav. Res. Ther.*, vol. 4, pp. 119–34.

ZUBIN, J. (1967), 'Classification of the behavior disorders', *Ann. Rev. Psychol.*, vol., 18, pp. 373–406.

Author Index

Author Index

Author Index

Subject Index

treatment of, 114–15, 152
Autohypnosis 129
Automated anxiety relief procedure 90–91
Automated desensitization 88, 211
Aversion therapy 95–106, 124, 203
  efficacy of 141–5, 152, 153
  experimental studies 187–92, 195
  in groups 96
  problems of 226–8
Aversive imagery therapy 105–6
Aversive stimuli 53, 98–9
Avoidance learning 31, 37, 41, 52–3
  use in aversion therapy 103–4, 144, 188–9
Awareness in operant conditioning 57, 201

Backward conditioning 35, 97
Belle indifférence 66
Bereavement 70, 71
  in childhood 62
Bibliotherapy 148
Blindness, hysterical 117–18
Body-rocking 64
Brain
  supposed source of mental disorder 14
  learning mechanisms in 39

CAD see Conditioned avoidance drive
CAR see Conditioned avoidance response
CER see Conditioned emotional response
Carbon dioxide inhalations 173
Cardiac responses 54, 79
Cat phobia, treatment of
  by anxiety relief technique 90–91
  by practical retraining 84
Causation of psychiatric disorders 13–15
Childhood
  aversive conditioning in 61–2
  bereavement in 62
  personality development in 18, 79, 80
  response to conflict in 65
  see also Infancy
Children

behaviour disorders in 73
generalization in 200
induced anxiety in 50
neurotic 116–17
phobias of 52, 83–4, 89, 131, 181–2, 226
  acquired by imitation 57
  psychotic 114–15 see also Autism
  relaxation difficulties of 223
Chlorpromazine 88, 107
Cigarette addiction
  treatment of 103, 106
  therapist's role in 209
Classical conditioning 27, 28–30, 34, 41
  compared with operant conditioning 33–4, 41, 42
  EEG patterns in 39
  fetishism induced by 72
  in aversion therapy 99
  in neurotic anxiety 50–52
  in psychosomatic disorders 68
  nature of response 33, 42
  optimal timing 35
Claustrophobia 216
  treatment of 84
  efficacy of 137
Client-centred therapy 22
Codeine phosphate 88
Cognitive processes 24, 79, 175, 176, 200, 202, 203, 217
Cognitive theory see Stimulus–stimulus theory
Compulsive disorders 202
  origin and maintenance of 217
  treatment of
    by aversion therapy 105
    by implosive therapy 111
Conceptual processes 56, 79
Conditioned anxiety response 50, 52, 96
Conditioned avoidance drive 41, 50
Conditioned avoidance response 31, 41–2, 52–3, 56–7, 63, 80, 156
Conditioned emotional response 50–51, 52, 56–7, 68
Conditioned inhibition 44, 120 see also Negative practice
Conditioning see Backward conditioning

Subject Index

Subject Index

Subject Index